Secret Potions, Elixirs & Concoctions

BOTANICAL & AROMATIC RECIPES
for MIND, BODY & SOUL

by Marie Anakee Miczak

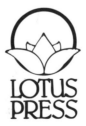

Published by:
Lotus Press
P.O. Box 325, Twin Lakes, WI 53181 USA

DISCLAIMER

This book is a reference work, not intended to diagnose, prescribe or treat. The information contained herein is in no way to be considered as a substitute for consultation with a licensed health care professional. It is designed to provide information on traditional uses of herbs and historical folklore remedies.

Cover Design: Irene Archer
Book Design & Layout: Irene Archer

For inquiries contact Lotus Press,
P.O. Box 325, Twin Lakes, WI 53181 USA
e-mail: lotuspress@lotuspress.com
web site: www.lotuspress.com
phone: (800) 824-6396

First Edition, 1999
Printed in the United States of America

Library of Congress Catalog Number: 98-75822
ISBN: 0-914955-45-4

Published by Lotus Press, P.O. Box 325, Twin Lakes, Wisconsin 53181

Contents

CHAPTER FOUR:
Skin & Body Care

CHAPTER FIVE:

CHAPTER SIX:

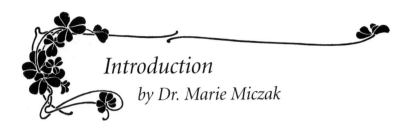

Introduction
by Dr. Marie Miczak

Not too long ago in man's seemingly distant past, we enjoyed an intimate relationship with the earth & all it produced. Each culture developed around its own use of herbs, fruits & other botanicals that later became their unique "ethnobotany", literally meaning the knowledge of plants used by a specific ethnic group for food, medicine & healing. Secret Potions, Elixirs & Concoctions offers an open door passage to the healing wisdom of ancient cultures from around the world. The combining of folklore & science makes for an enjoyable, easy to follow guide that you will delight to refer to again & again. In our busy world today, stress is perhaps the greatest stealer of good health, manifesting itself in hypertension, heart disease, anxiety attacks & gastrointestinal disturbances to name only a few. Therefore, whatever we can do to diminish this eroding factor in our lives will add not only years to our life, but life to our years!

As you move through the sampling of these exotic, time honored formulas, you will gain confidence in your proficiency to truly effect your own personal physical & mental status. From the soothing bath oils, to the delicately fragranced candles & sachets, you will find yourself wishing to share this fountain of joy with loved ones and fully understand what living well really means. The ingredients in these potions are not costly and there is no need to check yourself into an expensive spa to have them prepared. This wonderful world of scented earthly delights awaits with health benefits which are sure to last a lifetime!

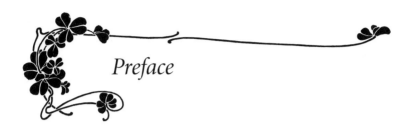

Preface

Dragons blood, bat wings, wine, spider webs and a pinch of ground mummy. Sounds like the quintessential brew, right? This is certainly most peoples view of a potion. Although it is true that in Medieval times some herbs were mixed with blood and that pulverized mummy was used in Victorian times for various complaints, the majority of concoctions passed down for generations were quite simple to prepare and used common ingredients. Likewise all of the ingredients used in this book may not be what you would think to use on the given applications but are safe and easily found in most supermarkets and health food stores.

In this day and age when it seems like a new breakthrough in medicine is found everyday, it's intriguing that people are looking to ancient teachings to heal themselves. Be it Aromatherapy, Ayurveda, Chinese, etc. people want the holistic option which these modalities offer instead of a one treatment fits all approach. During the Victorian period mainly in America, people started to put a large amount of faith into science and inventions. Herbal concoctions were now thrown into the Ùwives talesˆ and Ùsnake oilˆ category and subsequently looked down upon. Although a large amount of the elixirs produced and sold by salesmen were of no help or even harmful, many of the traditional healing practices brought over from immigrants' homelands were quite helpful. In lands where western medicine had not yet reached, people continued to treat their ailments and enrich their lives with homemade brews.

In this book you will find many recipes that were used long ago but remain beneficial even today. You will find them quite pleasing and easy to make as well. Since they are freshly made with no chemical preservatives, you are getting the full benefit of the herbs, botanicals, etc. that are essential in the healing process. Most concoctions are made in ten ways depending on the application in which it will be used and the type of herb/plant material if any. The easiest and probably most likely method you yourself already use frequently is the classic infusion. A more in depth explanation is found later on in the book but it simply entails pouring hot water over fresh or dried herbs. This works on delicate parts of a plant such as the flowers, buds and leaves. The plant material is steeped, strained off and the liquid is ingested as a simple tea. This and the decoction method was and still is heavily practiced in Chinese medicine. A patient would be given a prescription and be instructed to visit a herb shop to pick up the needed items. The Chinese way is to make a very strong brew which is taken in specific doses throughout the day or week.

Tinctures are another ancient form of extracting the healing effects of the herb or plant. Most tinctures are made by pouring alcohol over the plant matter and letting it sit for a period of time. Wine was often used but today vodka is recommended because of the high alcohol content. Syrups are also effective in treating various ailments. Being that it is made with honey, it helps cover any unpleasant taste that the herb might hold. First a decoction or infusion is made depending on the plant material and honey is added while the mixture is still hot. The ratio is 1:1 or uses equal parts honey to decoction/infusion. Both of these methods were used by European peoples to cure a great many illnesses such as coughs, sleeplessness, etc.

Other potions are made utilizing the hot/cold infusion, salve, compress, or poultice technique. If you look closely at many of the recipes you will see that they fall into one of the above categories or use some of the methods to make a more complex brew. Once you master the different ways of preparing concoctions it will be easier for you to formulate your own or add to the recipes in this book.

Another extremely important potion is perfume. Perfumery was not only used by peoples in ancient times to pleasantly scent their surroundings but also to heal and ward off what were thought to be air born diseases such as the plague. Herbs, spices, and botanicals were either burned, placed in water which was heated to carry the scent in the form of steam, or added to oils and other ingredients to form a perfume to be applied to the skin. Many cultures kept the art of perfumery and the essential oils used therein sacred. The Egyptians used cedarwood, frankincense, myrrh and other oils for embalming. The Greeks were probably the most lavish, using perfumes to scent their clothes, bedding, bodies, hair, walls, and more. Throughout Asia perfumes were turned into all sorts of incenses which were made and burned to release the potions into the air. Due to the rich history behind perfumery I thought it only fitting to teach you how to make your own... naturally. Today preparing your own fragrances is simple and you can choose from a large array of pure essential and fragrance oils. People have even found that wearing a single essential oil or note is quite pleasant.

There are so many potions and brews made by people all over the world. This book contains an exceptional sampling which I have personally experienced and modified for today's lifestyle. The ingredients are fairly easy to find and to help I have also included a resource area that contains mail order companies in which you can find many of the components needed for the recipes. Whether you are new to the world of potion making or a seasoned alchemist you will find these concoctions enjoyable to create, use and even give away as gifts. Why not benefit from what the past has to offer?

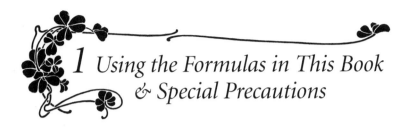

1 Using the Formulas in This Book & Special Precautions

Before preparing a formula in this book, be sure to look over the entire recipe first. Take the time to see if you have all the needed ingredients or if substitutions can be made to fit the materials you have on hand. With some of the more botanical based recipe make sure you have the freshest produce possible. If fresh fruits and/or vegetables are not available, use frozen with your last resort being canned. If you have no other choice than to use canned, wash thoroughly to remove any impurities such as sugar, salt etc. Fresh fruits and vegetables should if at all possible be organic. If this is not feasible make sure to use a special wash made for fruits and vegetables to remove any wax, colorants or chemicals that may be on the skin. Other botanical ingredients such as eggs, yogurt etc. should also be as extremely fresh for the best results. You will probably also notice once you flip through the recipes that they have a short shelf life and some must be kept in the refrigerator. This is due to the fact that there is no chemical preservatives added except for natural honey in a few. Once made most of the recipes should be used right away as they start to lose their effectiveness over time. Another threat to your creation is molds. If you see even a hint discard and start over again.

Choosing Herbs & Spices to Use

Fresh organic herbs are of course the best. Dried will also work well in many of the recipes found in this book. Many health food stores carry a wide variety of loose, dried herbs. You can also buy herbal teas and use the contents of the bag in your concoction. If you will be doing this make sure you find pure herbal teas that do not contain a large amount of fillers such as black tea, etc. Wild crafting is another way of obtaining herbs. Keep in mind though that plants next to roads can have high levels of lead and other chemicals from passing vehicular exhaust. Look also to see if the area in which you are picking herbs has been sprayed with pesticides or herbicides. Many park systems do this so try to find out before taking anything home. Growing your own herbs in a little garden is undoubtedly the best. Which ever route you choose, rinse your herbs well and spray with a fruit/vegetable wash if you think it's needed.

When it comes to spices the fresher the better. Look to make sure spices are vibrant in color and aroma. When ground spices are around too long they start to lose their healing qualities. Always make sure caps and lids are on tight and herbs are kept in a cool, dark place. Whole spices like cumin and coriander can be placed in pepper mills and freshly ground.

Equipment You may Need

Here is a list of items that will come in quite handy when making the recipes found in this book:
- Sauce pan and/or small pot
- Wooden, glass and/or ceramic bowls
- Blender or coffee grinder
- Small metal whisk

- Wooden spoons
- Chinese hat (sieve)
- Glass bottles and/or ceramic cups
- Measuring cups (wet and dry) and spoons
- Cheese cloth
- Mortar and pestle
- Wood chopping block

The All Important Patch Test

You will see references to a patch test throughout this book. Just what is it? Well, a patch test is taking a small amount of the formula you've just made and applying it to the skin on the inside of your arm. If after 24 hours no rash or tenderness appears, then the recipe is safe to use. If even a hint of irritation shows up do not continue use and discard. If you do find you have a reaction that persists go to a dermatologist or doctor as soon as possible. Do this with each and every recipe in this book. It is an extremely important step that should not be skipped.

Other Words of Caution

Just like with OTC products you buy, keep all formulas out of the reach of children. Make sure you clearly mark the concoction you just made and are now storing in the refrigerator. A child unknowingly could mistake it for a beverage or food item, ingest a bit and become ill. I highly suggest getting a pack of peel and stick labels and a black marking pen. Cover formula containers with plastic wrap and stick on a label. Write the recipes name and date of preparation. This way other family members may not take it for moldy food and toss it! Also you can keep an eye on the date to make sure you're not storing it too long.

Lore

~~~ ~~~ ~~~

Rosemary was burned by people in the Middle Ages to drive away evil spirits and to protect them from contracting the plague.

In Medieval times it was quite common for young adults to be seen standing in the light of the full moon with a rope of garlic tied around their necks. Why? To get rid of acne of course...

The word "shaman" was derived from a word in the Tungusic language of Siberia. This is a place where the classical form of shamanism can be found still in practice.

One of the earliest medical physicians to be discovered by archaeologists is a man named Imhotep who was a much consulted adviser to the Pharaoh of Egypt. In that time physicians were also considered priests and magicians.

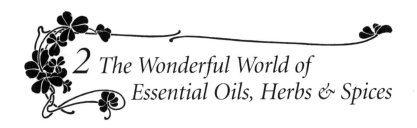

2 The Wonderful World of Essential Oils, Herbs & Spices

Below are easy to use charts describing herbs, essential Aromatherapy oils and spices.

Aromatherapy Essential Oils:

There are over 300 different Aromatherapy oils which have been extracted from a variety of sources such as plants, fruits, flowers, and barks. Essential oils not only serve as scents, but can also work to heal and soothe the body and soul. Remember to look for pure essential oils which are steamed distilled, not fragrance oils which are fake reproductions. They do not hold the same properties and most likely are chemically manufactured. Some of the recipes in this book do call for fragrance oils however, in small amounts and purely for aroma enhancement. Some examples are honeysuckle, strawberry, musk, etc.

Essential Oil Chart

These are easy to find essential oils sure to be key additions to your collection.

BERGAMOT (*Citrus bergamia*):
Aroma: Cool yet spicy citrus. **Origins:** Ancient Asia and named after a city in Italy. **Main attributes:** Uplifting and an aphrodisiac, bergamot is a wonderful antidepressant and analgesic. Works well for acne and other skin conditions and colds. **Safety note:** May be irritating in high amounts.

CEDARWOOD (*Cedrus atlantica*)**Aroma:** Spicy and resinous. **Origins:** The Algerian mountains and heavily used by the Egyptians. **Main attributes:** Held as a extremely sacred essential oil by the Egyptians you will find it stimulating yet relaxing. Great for acne and other skin eruptions/infections. May be used in room diffusers for colds, stress and tension relief. **Safety note:** A good idea to be avoided by pregnant women.

LAVENDER (*Lavandula augustfolia*):
Aroma: Earthy and green. **Origins:** Mediterranean. **Main attributes:** Works wonders to calm nerves and help with sleep problems. Lavender is an extremely important essential oil and I highly recommend having some on hand at all times. An antidepressant, nervine, and stress reliever. Great for acne, burns and other skin conditions.

ORANGE (*Citrus aurantium*):
Aroma: True orange scent. **Origins:** The Far East. **Main attributes:** A truly uplifting oil. Known for it's antidepressant and calming effects on the body. **Safety note:** May be irritating to the skin in large amounts and not to be used before going to sleep.

ROSE (*Rosa centifolia*):
Aroma: Rich and sensuous. **Origins:** Thought to have been a native to Asia but known for it's use in Europe. **Main**

attributes: The people of the Middle Ages adored it and it is still the symbol of love with good cause. A highly effective antidepressant and aphrodisiac you will find it worth every penny. Wonderful for mature skin and various epidermal problems. Great in a diffuser to help remedy allergies and respiratory problems.

PATCHOULI *(Pogostemon cablin):*
Aroma: Woody and sweet. **Origins:** Islands of Asia. **Main attributes:** Use to help balance your mind and body as it has been shown to reduce stress and anxiety. You will find it superb on skin conditions such as acne, wind burn, wrinkles etc. Does well as an insect repellent also. **Safety note:** May sting if allowed to enter open cuts. Try to use only on unbroken skin.

PEPPERMINT *(Mentha piperata):*
Aroma: Strong and sweet. **Origins:** Not known, thought to be found world-wide. **Main attributes:** An extremely effective antidepressant and tension reliever. Use it in a diffuser to relieve colds and other respiratory problems. It also has an antiseptic quality that makes it suited to cleaning non wood surfaces. This oil does tend to take over so use it in small amounts and not before bed unless in a chest rub. **Safety note:** People with sensitive skin should pass on this oil and high amounts should not be used.

SANDALWOOD *(Santalum album):*
Aroma: Vary warming, spicy and woody. **Origins:** Asia. **Main attributes:** Highly euphoric and an aphrodisiac it also helps a plethora of skin conditions such as acne, wind burn, etc. Also helps relieve nausea and nervous tension.

TEA TREE *(Melaleuca alternifolia):*
Aroma: Green. **Origins:** Australia. **Main attributes:** Long used by the aborigines of Australia, it has a broad antiseptic and anti-fungal quality that lends itself well to skin disorders such as acne, athlete's foot fungal infections, burns and more. Great for use in cleaning non wood surfaces to disinfect without harsh chemicals. **Safety note:** Some people with sensitive skin may find it irritating.

YLANG YLANG *(Cananga ordorata):*
Aroma: Very unique and floral. **Origin:** Islands of Asia. **Main attributes:** A superb oil to use on the hair and scalp. Helps with many skin problems such as insect bites, oily skin, acne etc. Also known to reduce depression, sleeplessness, stress and other nervine problems. It has long been considered a strong aphrodisiac. **Safety note:** In large amounts it may cause nausea and headaches. Can irritate the skin as well in large amounts. A few drops is all you really need with this essential oil.

Herbal Chart

More and more people are looking at what may be growing right in their own backyard to heal their ailments. Before buying herbs in dry/fresh form take the time to look over this chart of the most common ones. Just like with prescription and OTC drugs, you can suffer side affects and/or overdoses. Due to this I have included safety information so that you can make a wiser decision on using a particular herb.

CHAMOMILE (Roman: *Chamaemelum nobile*) & (German: *Matricaria recutita*):
Origins: (Roman) southern and western Europe. (German) Europe and parts of Asia. Keep in mind there are many species and to use the ones I have listed for the most benefits. **Main**

attributes: Holds sedative, anti-nausea, nerve sedative, calming and anti-inflammatory capabilities. May be used in infusions, tinctures, diffusers and ointments. **Safety note:** People who are pregnant should avoid this herb. May cause irritation for people with sensitive skin.

DANDELION (*Taraxacum officinale*):
Origins: Europe. **Main attributes:** Contains many vitamins and minerals including A, B, C, D, iron and others. Strong liver tonic and diuretic. Many people view this plant as a nuisance weed but when you start to look at all the healing properties you may wish more would grow. The root can be put in a tincture or decocted and the leaves can be used in salads, juices, or infusions.

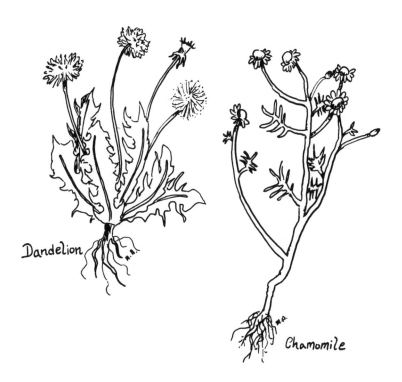

Dandelion

Chamomile

GOLDENSEAL (*Hydrastis canadensis*):
Origins: Americas. **Main attributes**: A tonic herb that helps to aid digestion and excretion of chemical build-up in the system. May also help with the symptoms of PMS and menopause. Works well in the form of capsules, tinctures, and infusion teas. Traditionally used by native American peoples of the Iroquois tribe for liver and heart problems, digestion as well as whooping cough. **Safety note**: A uterine stimulant, it would be wise to avoid if pregnant. If you have high blood pressure do not ingest this herb. Also do not attempt to eat the plant raw.

HONEYSUCKLE (*Lonicera spp.*):
Origins: Europe and Asia. **Main attributes**: A diuretic, laxative when taken internally. Topically it can help soothe and smooth the skin. Works well in the form of a syrup or tea infusion for the flowers. The stems can be turned into a decoction and used in many applications. **Safety note:** Never use berries that show up on some species, they are poisonous.

MINT (*Mentha spp.*):
Origins: Almost worldwide. **Main attributes:** Has antidepressant, sedative, relaxing quality. Also helps with digestion and may be taken as a tea after meals. Best used in infusions, tinctures, ointments and compresses. **Safety note:** May irritate sensitive skin.

PURPLE CONEFLOWER (*Echinacea spp.*):
Origins: Americas. **Main attributes:** An antibiotic and immune system stimulant the root can be used in capsules, decoctions, massage oils and tinctures. Long used by the native Americans for snake bite, colds, wounds etc. it has now been found to help stimulate the immune system to ward off colds and shorten existing ones. **Safety note:** Can cause nau-

sea and dizziness in large amounts.

ROSEMARY (*Rosmarinus officinalis*):
Origins: Mediterranean. **Main attributes:** Has astringent, nervine and diuretic qualities. Helps to stimulate blood flow when applied topically. Herb may be infused, made into a tincture, hair rinse, cream or compress. **Safety note:** People who have high blood pressure, seizures or who are pregnant should pass on this herb.

RED CLOVER (*Trifolium pratense*):
Origins: Europe and the Mediterranean. **Main attributes:** Holds anti-inflammatory and diuretic properties. Works well for skin problems topically in the form of compresses, ointments, baths, creams and tinctures. Can also be used in a diffuser for cold and cough relief.

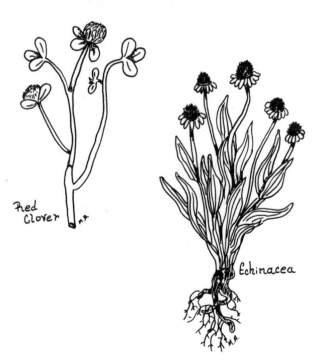

Red Clover

Echinacea

SAGE (*Salvia spp.*):
Origins: Native to Europe and the Mediterranean depending on the species. **Main attributes:** Said to have beneficial affects on the memory and power of recollection. It has astringent and antibiotic qualities as well. Works well in infusions, tincture, hair tonics and compresses. Decoctions can be made from the root. Native American people used it for healing sores and colds while the Chinese used it as a tonic for heart and liver conditions. **Safety note:** People who have epileptic seizures or are prone to them and pregnant/nursing women should steer clear of this herb.

VIOLET (*Viola odorata*):
Origins: Europe and some areas of Asia as it now grows almost world wide. **Main attributes:** Due to it's antiseptic and anti-inflammatory qualities it makes it quite effective in treating various skin conditions such as eczema and acne. Both the leaves and flowers can be used in a variety of ways with the most common being infusions, creams, syrups, tinctures and poultices. **Safety note:** Be careful not to use in high doses as it may cause nausea and even vomiting in some cases.

Spice Chart

Spices have been traditionally used by people practicing Ayurvedic medicine in India for more than five thousand years. It is of course only a small part of this complex art but an important one. Today you can mix spices with herbs, essential oils, etc., to make wonderful, healing concoctions. Use the chart below to help with your formulations.

ALLSPICE (*Pimenta dioica*):
Origins: South America and West Indies. **Main attributes:** Relaxation and antiseptic qualities. Great if used in a diffuser

for respiratory problems and tension relief. **Safety note**: Use in very small amounts and highly diluted on the skin. May cause irritation to sensitive skin.

CINNAMON (*Cinnamon spp.*):
Origins: African and Asian Islands. **Main attributes**: Works well for immune system problems such as colds. Contains antiseptic properties. Use in decoctions, room mists, and tinctures. In Chinese medicine it was used to help with circulation and bring blood to the extremities as well as lack of appetite and menstrual pains. **Safety note**: May be irritating to sensitive skin. Never use in a bath. Avoid use if pregnant or have a high fever.

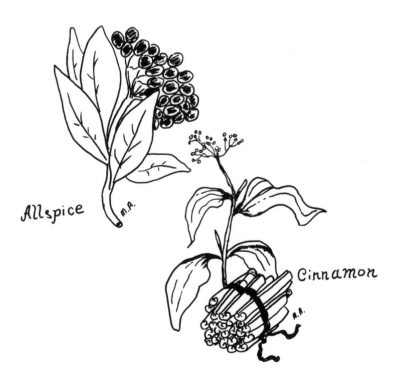

Allspice

Cinnamon

CLOVE (*Syzygium aromaticum*):
Origins: Indonesian Islands. **Main attributes**: It's antiseptic, antibiotic and antiviral properties makes it perfect for room mists, diffusers, household natural cleaners and more. Can also help skin conditions such as acne, fungal infections, burns etc. Use in steam facials and warm compresses. **Safety note:** People with sensitive skin should be careful with cloves and use in a very diluted form.

CUMIN (*Cuminum cyminum*):
Origins: Egypt. **Main attributes**: Cumin usually found as one of the ingredients of any good curry actually has antiseptic, bactericidal, and even an aphrodisiac effect on the body. Works well for circulation problems, toxic build up in the system, headaches and more. Place in diffusers for a spicy, calming affect. **Safety note:** Avoid heavy use during pregnancy.

GINGER (*Zingiber officinalis*):
Origins: Asia. **Main attributes**: A strong circulatory stimulant it can help with hair growth and aid cold hands and feet. Helps to relieve nausea. Use in the form of a decoction, tincture, or cream. **Safety note**: Use in small amounts.

MUSTARD (*Brassica nigra*):
Origins: Europe, Africa, and parts of Asia. **Main attributes:** Holds antiseptic and antimicrobial properties. Traditionally used for colds, coughs, etc. **Safety note:** Use in small amounts and only in a poultice.

NUTMEG (*Myristica fragrans*):
Origins: Bande Islands. **Main attributes:** Helps to relieve the feeling of nausea, stomach upset, loss of appetite, diarrhea and other gastric problems. Can be used in decoctions, capsules, and essential oil blends. In Ayurvedic medicine it is

mixed with ginger to help calm the stomach. **Safety note:** Do not take in large doses. May cause heart palpitations, delirium and even convulsions.

TURMERIC (*Curcuma longa*):
Origins: Asia. **Main attributes:** Also used in curry powder it has many beneficial qualities. Diuretic, bactericidal, anti-inflammatory to name a few. Works well on muscular and joint problems. Mix into creams and ointments for relief of minor aches and pains. Also may be used in a poultice. **Safety note**: Do not use if you have sensitive skin.

STAR ANISE (*Illicium verum*):
Origins: China and Asian Islands. **Main attributes:** Helps to aid respiratory problems such as coughs, colds, aches, etc. Use in poultices and creams. **Safety note:** Avoid if pregnant and use in small amounts.

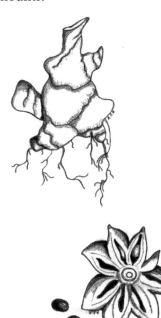

Quotes and Ancient Proverbs

Among thorns grow roses.
— Italian Proverb

Cheerfulness is the very flower of health.
— Japanese Proverb

"Speak to the earth, and it shall teach thee."
— Bible, Job 12:8

*"The best and most beautiful things
in the world cannot be seen or even touched.
They must be felt with the heart."*
— Helen Keller

"Man is the only animal that blushes. Or needs to."
— Mark Twain

*"Glowing moments of peaceful reflection kindle
the growth of our minds and spirits."*
— Anonymous

*"Life would be infinitely happier if we could
only be born at the age of eighty and
gradually approach eighteen.*
— Mark Twain

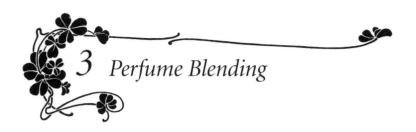

3 Perfume Blending

Perfume making is an ancient art most likely started by the Egyptians. Through the mixing of essential and fragrance oils you can make totally unique and natural perfumes suited to you and you alone. Feel free to experiment and make new blends. One thing to remember is to strive to keep it as simple as possible. Some of the most aromatic blends come from two or three oil combinations. Always keep in mind what note category the essential oil falls in. Example; Lavender is a top note, meaning it will be the first aroma you smell in a perfume blended with it. It is also the first oil to evaporate when applied to your skin. Patchouli on the other hand is a base note, meaning it is the last fragrance you will notice. It is most likely to be left on your skin when the top and middle notes have disappeared. Use the charts below to find out what oils will complement each other and blend well.

Essential Aromatherapy Oil Blending Chart

Top Notes:

BERGAMOT: Blends well with Jasmine, Neroli, Chamomile, Patchouli, other citrus oils & most florals.

CORIANDER: Blends well with Sandalwood, Bergamot, Neroli & most florals.

GRAPEFRUIT: Blends well with Orange, Cinnamon & other citrus oils.

LAVENDER: Blends well with Geranium & most citrus oils.

LEMON: Blends well with Lavender, Cedarwood & Ylang Ylang.

ORANGE: (sweet) Blends well with Cinnamon, Cloves, Nutmeg, Ylang Ylang & Sandalwood.

PETITGRAIN: Blends well with Lavender, Rosemary, bitter & sweet Orange, Jasmine & most spicy oils.

TEA TREE : Blends well with Lavender.

Top to Middle Notes & Middle Note Oils:

CHAMOMILE: Blends well with Jasmine, Rose, Lavender.

CLARY SAGE: Blends well with Lavender, Orange, Sandalwood & most florals.

JUNIPER: Blends well with Bergamot, Sandalwood, Rosemary.

LEMONGRASS: Blends well with Lavender, Rose, Geranium.

LEMON BALM: Blends well with Rose, Lavender, Neroli, Geranium.

MARJORAM: Blends well with Lavender, Bergamot, Rosemary.

PALMAROSA: Blends well with Rosewood, Sandalwood, Cedarwood & most florals.

THYME: Blends well with Bergamot, Lavender, Lemon Balm, Pine.

Middle to Base Notes & Base Note Oils:

CYPRESS: Blends well with Juniper, Bergamot, Lemon & Pine.

CEDARWOOD: Blends well with Bergamot, Juniper, Neroli, Sandalwood & Jasmine.

GINGER: Blends well with Lavender & Orange.

NUTMEG: Blends well with Cloves, Orange, Cinnamon & Rosemary.

PATCHOULI: Blends well with Sandalwood, Cedarwood, Rose, Jasmine, Lemon & Ylang Ylang.

PEPPERMINT: Blends well with Lavender, Rose & Rosemary.

PINE: Blends well with Lavender, Sage & Rosemary.

SANDALWOOD: Blends well with Rose, Jasmine, Ylang Ylang & most woody oils.

YLANG YLANG: Blends well with Sandalwood, Orange, Lemon, Neroli, Bergamot & Jasmine.

Fragrance Oil Blending Chart

Top Note Oils:

BERGAMOT: Blends well with most florals, Violet & Geranium.

LEMON VERBENA: Blends well with Lemon & other citrus oils.

LIME: Blends well with most florals, Orange & Geranium.

LEMON: Blends well with Rose, Benzoin & most citrus oils.

MANDARIN ORANGE: Blends well with Rose, Ylang Ylang, most spicy & fruit oils.

Top to Middle Notes & Middle Note Oils:

ALMOND: Blends well with Nutmeg, Cloves, & Vanilla.

CARNATION: Blends well with Heliotrope, Musk & most spicy oils.

CHERRY: Blends well with most citrus & fruit oils, Vanilla & Almond.

COCONUT: Blends well with Ylang Ylang, Vanilla, Banana & Gardenia.

CLOVES: Blends well with Peppermint, most spicy & citrus oils.

GARDENIA: Blends well with Musk, Heliotrope & fruit oils.

HONEYSUCKLE: Blends well with Musk, floral & woody oils.

JASMINE: Blends well with Strawberry, Musk, Rose & citrus oils.

LILAC: Blends well with Rose, Violet & Musk.

LIME: Blends well with most floral & citrus oils, Lavender & Rosemary.

MANDARIN ORANGE: Blends well with most spicy oils, Rose, Jasmine & Ylang Ylang.

MANGO: Blends well with Vanilla, Coconut, Banana & Musk.

PEACH: Blends well with Violet, Vanilla & Jasmine.

ROSE: Blends well with Musk, Orange blossoms, Cassie, spicy oils & Jasmine.

VIOLET: Blend well with spicy oils, Musk, Clary sage, & Strawberry.

Middle to Base Notes & Base Note Oils:

BANANA: Blends well with most fruit oils, Vanilla & Coconut.

CEDARWOOD: Blends well with Neroli, Rose, Sandalwood, Rosewood, Ylang Ylang & floral oils.

CINNAMON: Blends well with Violet, Orange, Mandarin, & Benzoin.

FRANKINCENSE: Blends well with Lavender, Pine, Mimosa, Cinnamon, Black pepper & other spicy oils.

HELIOTROPE: Blends well with Orange, Violet & Carnation.

MUSK: Blends well with most florals & Vanilla.

MYRRH: Blends well with: Lavender, Pine, Geranium, woody oils & mint oils.

VANILLA: Blends well with Bergamot, Ylang Ylang, Cloves,

Lavandin & Patchouli.

Note that fragrance oils are only used in recipes in this book for aroma enhancement. Fragrance and essential aromatherapy oils can be mixed together.

As you can see, it would be quite easy for you to create a wonderful personal scent just by using the charts. If you need more guidance though, try some of the superb recipes below.

Amorousness Perfume

20 drops of Sandalwood essential oil
10 drops of Rose essential / fragrance oil
5 drops of Musk fragrance oil
10 drops of Jasmine essential oil
1 teaspoon of jojoba or sweet almond oil
¼ teaspoon of honey

This may sound a bit strange, but the results are simply magical. This blend also gets better with time! If you were wondering, the honey acts as a natural preservative. You may never want to buy perfumes from the department store again after trying this.

Oriental Song

¼ teaspoon of ground Cinnamon or 5 drops of essential / fragrance oil
5 drops of Musk fragrance oil
2 drops of Lemongrass essential oil
1 teaspoon jojoba or sweet almond oil

This is a wonderful, light perfume. Its best to let it sit in a dark, cool place for about a week before using. The Lemongrass adds an uplifting quality.

Silver Moon

10 drops of Jasmine essential / fragrance oil.

3 drops of Sandalwood essential oil

1 to 2 drops of Vanilla oil or pure extract

1 teaspoon jojoba or sweet almond oil

With Jasmine, known as the queen of the night, as the main note in this perfume it's perfect for an evening out and an evening to remember.

Sea Zephyr

10 drops of Orange essential oil

½ teaspoon of sea salt

2 drops of Neroli essential oil

1 teaspoon jojoba or sweet almond oil

The salt serves more for show than scent, so don't worry if it doesn't dissolve. It does add just a bit of the sea to the blend though. The perfume comes out just as nice without it, so if you haven't any around, don't fret.

Tropical Sun

5 drops Cherry fragrance oil

5 drops Peach fragrance oil

1 or 2 drops of Strawberry fragrance oil

½ teaspoon of pure Banana or Coconut extract

1 teaspoon jojoba or sweet almond oil

Mix all ingredients together and let sit a day or so before using to let scents mingle. The banana or coconut extract may separate from the oil, so shake very well before applying. It is a good rule of thumb to put all perfumes you make in glass bottles. The essential oils are very potent and may leach from plastic ones.

If you were wondering what goes into a professionally blended perfume, I have a few well known names and their aromatic makeup. As you can see they are quite complicated and utilize many oils.

Eternity by Calvin Klein

Top Notes: Mixture of Citruses
Middle Notes: Lily of the Valley, Lilac, Jasmine, Rose, Carnation and Violet.
Base Notes: Sandalwood, Musk.

Opium

Top Notes: Orange, Bay.
Middle Notes: Carnation, Rose, Ylang Ylang, Cinnamon, Peach, Jasmine, Orris/Iris.
Base Notes: Amber, Benzoin, Vanilla, Sandalwood, Patchouli, Musk.

Gio

Top Note: Hyacinth
Middle Notes: Rose, Jasmine, Neroli, Ylang Ylang, Iris/Orris, Cloves, Gardenia, Peach.
Base Notes: Sandalwood, Vanilla, Amber.

Pheromone

Top Notes: A mixture of Barks, Seeds and Flower scents along with Jasmine.
Middle Notes: Lotus flowers, Neroli, Ylang Ylang, Iris, Rosemary, Tonka extract.
Base Notes: Patchouli, Oakmoss, Sandalwood.

Not all commercial fragrances contain a great number of

aromatic oils. Once again simpler sometimes is better. This is true of Jivago, Anne Pliska, and Gardenia Passion which only contain around seven scents as opposed to Perfume Must de Cartier and Sung which use over twenty.

In the perfume business blended perfumes are given categories with the most common being Floral, Oriental, and Fruity. The oils are also given scent classifications such as green, woody, sweet, fruity, floral, fresh, spicy, powdery, delicious, tropical, etc. Here is an example of how a perfume is formulated using these groupings.

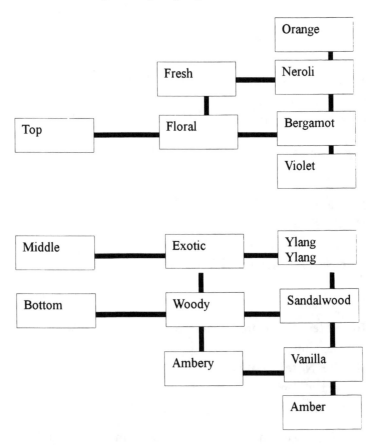

You too can use this form of grouping to create your own scents. Instead of just sticking to the top notes, middle notes, etc. you can get more elaborate by organizing all the woody notes together, floral notes, and so on to form a special blend. Here is a list of the basic scent categories and the oils that fall into them.

Floral: Rose, jasmine, violet, orange blossom/neroli, lily of the valley, narcissus.

Fruity: Orange, peach, lemon, cassie, bergamot, pineapple, mango, coconut, mint, freesia.

Spicy: Ginger, cinnamon, cloves, ylang ylang, coriander.

Woody: Cedarwood, sandalwood, pine, amber, tuberose, frankincense.

Green: Coriander, hyacinth, lavender, rosemary, bay, sage, chamomile.

Exotic: Musk, ylang ylang, gardenia, vanilla.

Keep in mind that this information does not just apply to perfumes. You can use the charts to help concoct blends for massage oils, bath crystals, incense and more.

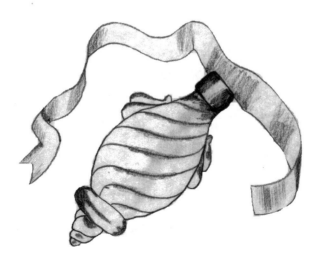

The Secret Language of Flowers

In early Victorian times there were of course no telephones and postage stamps were quite expensive, so people sent one another flowers. Not just any flowers but bouquets that held special meanings to the recipient and sender. You can carry on this practice the next time you send flowers to a friend or family member. Choose from the flowers below that best represent your wishes and/or thoughts.

Calendula: Despair, sorrow, many cares, and much heartache.

Carnation: Remorse, refusal, and sadness.

Chrysanthemums: Friendship, happiness, truth, and love.

Gladiolus: Strength and readiness.

Lily Of The Valley: Newfound happiness and purity.

Rose: Love, beauty, and utmost devotion.

Sweet Pea: Devotion, love and separation.

Violet: Modesty and steadfastness.

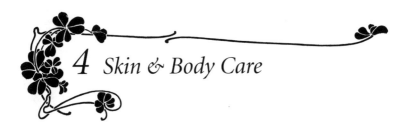

4 Skin & Body Care

A great number of posh spas are now using "natural" and "botanical based" treatments. Some are even prepared fresh on site. The problem comes with the fact that many people do not have the funds to pay the ridiculous fees charged by some establishments. If they are able to pay, they can only afford to be pampered once or twice a year on special occasions perhaps. Some treatments need to be applied on a regular basis before you start to notice a real difference. Lastly, many people don't feel like or have the time to trudge into a spa for the whole day. To remedy this, many spas and cosmetic companies are now producing and marketing products to use at home. Unfortunately these products can be quite expensive as well and do not use 100% pure and natural ingredients. The only real way to know exactly what your putting on your skin is to make the product yourself. Of course you can not make everything at home, but little by little you will find yourself replacing store bought items with the sensuously pleasing ones found in this book.

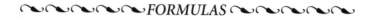

FORMULAS

✿ BODY CARE

Honeysuckle Body Elixir

　　1 Cup fresh honeysuckle flowers
　　2 Cups spring or distilled water
　　1 teaspoon pure vanilla extract

In a small pot bring water to a boil, reduce heat to very low and add flowers. Turn heat off completely after 10 minutes. Cover and let stand on stove for 5 hours. When done strain off all plant material and place in a clean glass bottle. Use as a all over body mist or in clay masks. Keep all unused portions refrigerated and for no longer than a week.

Variations:

Try these recipes for your specific skin needs.

Gentle:

　　1 Cup of fresh rose petals or ½ dried
　　1 Cup of water

Rose is extremely gentle for sensitive skin. Use after a bath for a real treat.

Refreshing:

　　2 Tablespoons of lemon zest
　　1 Cup of water
　　1 teaspoon of vanilla extract

This formula works great in the morning after a shower to help wake up your senses.

Moisturizing:

1 Cup of fresh rose petals or ½ dried
1 Cup of water
1 teaspoon of banana extract
5 drops rose essential oil (optional)

Placing body elixirs in mist bottles will make it easier for you to use and enjoy.

Amazon Rain

4 Cups spring or distilled water
½ teaspoon honey
10 drops of coconut fragrance oil or 2 teaspoons coconut extract
½ teaspoon pure vanilla extract
5 drops of jasmine essential oil

Mix all ingredients together and place in a spray bottle taking care to shake it well before using. This is a wonderful, lightly scented mist that you can use as you exercise or after a day of outdoor fun. Keep all unused portions in the refrigerator and no longer than a week.

Cleopatra's Milk Bath

2 Cups of dry milk powder
½ Cup cornstarch
5 drops of sandalwood essential oil
½ teaspoon of pure vanilla extract
one square piece of cheese cloth

Mix all ingredients in a small bowl until well incorporated. Place half the recipe in the middle of the cheese cloth square, forming a mound. Bring the four corners together and tie with a piece of string. Run a hot bath and place bag under running water. When bath has cooled to a comfortable temperature, gently squeeze the bag. At the end of the bath, quickly shower off any milk residue.

Shanghai Salts

> 2 Cups cornstarch
> 1 Cup rice flour
> ½ teaspoon ground cinnamon
> ¼ Tablespoon ground dried ginger
> 1 Tablespoon cloves
> 10 drops essential orange oil
> ½ Cup Epsom salts
> 1 to 2 drops of yellow food coloring

Place all ingredients in a blender and mix well. Put 4 tablespoons in hot running water. Spicy and exotic, this is sure to become one of your favorite treats. Small candy jars with lids make the perfect containers. Store in a cool, dry place.

Crystal Salts

> ½ Cup of sea salt
> 1 Cup of baking soda
> ½ Cup Epsom salts
> 20 drops of lemongrass essential oil
> A few drops of red food coloring (optional)

Mix all together well until completely blended. Place in a pretty glass bottle using a natural sea shell from the shore as measuring scoop. Keep in a cool, dry place.

Love Bath

> 1 Cup freshly picked rose petals
> ½ Cup dried milk

10 drops rose essential oil
1 cheese cloth square

Combine all ingredients together in a bowl and transfer
to the cheese cloth forming a mound in the center. Bring the
four corners together and tie with a piece of string. Run the
bath water steaming hot and place bag under running water.
When bath is at a comfortable temperature, take the bag and
squeeze it a couple of times before entering.

Peppermint Candy Soak

2 Cups of spring or distilled water
½ Cup of loose peppermint tea or 2 tea bags
½ Cup Epsom salts
10 drops of peppermint essential oil

Bring water to a boil and add tea. Turn heat off and let
steep for 1 or 2 hours depending on the strength you want.
Remove tea bags and place all ingredients in a blender until
incorporated. Clean glass bottles with corks or tops work best
as containers. When ready to use, give the bottle a good shake
and pour in as much as you desire to bath water. Store all
unused portions in your refrigerator for no more than 2
weeks. Great for sore, tired feet as well. Very invigorating, so
don't use at night unless you're going dancing!

Mermaid's Lagoon

1 Cup of Epsom salts
1 Cup of coarse sea salt
10 drops frangipani fragrance oil or essential oil
10 drops of blue food coloring

Combine all ingredients well and place in a container
with a lid. Epsom salts do have the tendency to evaporate.

Light and refreshing this will quickly become one of your favorite indulgences.

Star Burst

> 1 Cup of Epsom salts
> 1 Cup of baking soda
> 20 drops of strawberry fragrance oil
> 10 drops of yellow food coloring
> 1 vanilla bean, split open

Mix first four ingredients together in a large bowl. The reason this recipe calls for yellow food coloring instead of red to produce a pink color is because these salts are supposed to smell like delicious star fruit. Unfortunately star fruit scents aren't easily accessible so strawberry will suffice. Place the mixture in a clean container putting the vanilla bean straight down the center. With time the vanilla bean will add a warm touch to your Star Burst salts. Let cure 2 weeks before using. Store in cool, dry place in a container with a tight fitting lid.

Queen of the Night Body Butter

> 8 Tablespoon jojoba or sweet almond oil (base)
> 1 teaspoon vitamin E
> 1 Tablespoon margarine
> 10 drops of jasmine essential oil
> 3 drops of vanilla essential oil
> ½ teaspoon of honey
> 1 teaspoon natural bees wax

Place all ingredients in a saucepan. Mix until completely melted and combined. Turn heat off and pour into a clean jar. Cover and place in the refrigerator. You may need to blend it a bit before using. A little goes a long way.

❧ COMPLETE BODY TREATMENT

With this set of treatments you can turn your home into a lavish spa for a day. Be sure to look over all the steps first before proceeding and make adjustments to the concoctions depending on your skin type.

Almond Body Polisher

4 Tablespoons baking soda
½ Cup white corn meal
10 natural almonds
1 Tablespoon almond extract

In a coffee grinder place almonds and pulse until ground well. The same can be done in a blender. Blend all ingredients together and store in the refrigerator until ready to use.

Rose Water Clay Mask

1 Cup of rose Body Elixir
5 drops rose essential oil (optional)
Enough dry clay to make a thick mask
1 teaspoon sweet almond or olive oil

Stir together well and store in a clean container. Place in the refrigerator until ready to use.

Cherry Bath Oil

4 Tablespoons olive oil
2 Tablespoons canola oil
2 Tablespoons sweet almond oil
½ teaspoon vitamin E
10 drops of cherry fragrance oil

In a small bowl mix all ingredients together. Keep refrigerated until ready to use.

Violet Body Splash

2 Cups fresh violet flowers
3 Cups spring or distilled water
½ teaspoon vanilla extract

Heat water to a boil. Add flower petals and simmer for 15 minutes covered. Turn heat off and let sit 1 hour. Pour into a glass container or ceramic cup and keep refrigerated until ready to use. Strain off plant material and add vanilla extract. If fresh violets are not in season use one of the other Body Elixirs in this book.

Step one:

Wet skin before applying the Almond Body Scrub. Spread on Scrub and gently massage in a circular motion to remove dead skin. Rinse off with warm water.

Step two:

Apply Rose Water Clay Mask to arms, legs, thighs etc. keeping in mind to avoid sensitive skin areas. Spread on a thin layer and let dry for about 20 minutes.

Step three:

Draw a warm bath and add the Cherry Bath Oil. When water is a comfortable temperature enter and soak until clay can be wiped off easily with a wash cloth.

Step four:

Douse yourself quickly with the Violet Body Splash. If you like you can use the Queen of the Night Body Butter for an even more moisturizing effect.

Note: Remember to always do a patch test.

ࣔ FACIAL FORMULAS

Youth In a Bottle

10 drops rose essential oil
10 drops neroli essential oil
10 drops orange essential oil
1 Cup spring water

Place ingredients in order listed taking care to use a very clean glass bottle. Shake well before applying to freshly washed skin. Please do not substitute any of the essential oils for fragrance oils. The affect of this treatment will not be the same.

Rose Oil Rejuvenator

10 drops rose essential oil
2 Tablespoons sweet almond oil
3 drops geranium essential oil

Mix well. Keep in a glass bottle in the refrigerator. Use as spot treatment for wrinkles and/or fine lines or as an all over face moisturizer. Do not use around the eyes.

Rose Facial Steam

½ Cup fresh rose petals or ¼ Cup dried
5 drops rose essential oil (optional)
½ teaspoon vanilla extract
Enough water to fill a large bowl

Using a tea kettle bring water to a rolling boil. Place a large bowl on a hard, flat surface like a table. Add petals, extract and essential oil. Drape a bath towel over your head and pour water into the bowl. Move your face as close as possible to the steam without burning yourself. If steam is too hot, let it cool a bit. Stay under the towel for about 20 to 30 minutes. Use no more then once a week.

European Milk Cleanser

>   2 Cups dried milk
>   1 vanilla bean (optional)
>   5 drops of lavender

Mix together and place in a container with a lid. Store in a dark, cool place. To use, moisten a small amount in your hand with water and smooth over face and neck. Use the balls of your fingers to make small circular motions over your skin. Rinse well with warm water. Not only will this cleanse your skin but also help even out your complexion.

Strawberry Yogurt Mask

>   ¼ Cup plain yogurt
>   3 fresh strawberries
>   3 drops of lavender essential oil

Remove the green leaves and stems from the strawberry. Using a fork smash it until it is a fine pulp. You can also use a blender or small food processor. Mix in yogurt and essential oil. Smooth over clean skin and leave on for 15 to 20 minutes. Wash off with warm water. You will find this mask quite soothing and cooling to the skin. Discard any unused portions.

Cleansing Rice Mask

>   ¼ Cup rice milk
>   Enough clay to make a thick paste
>   3 drops of geranium

In a cup or bowl combine all ingredients and mix well.

Spread a thin layer over cleaned skin. Leave on for 15 to 20 minutes or until dry. Remove with warm water.

Ginger After Shave for Men

½ teaspoon fresh ginger
5 drops lavender
½ teaspoon honey
1 Cup water

Bring water to a boil. Reduce heat and add ginger. Simmer for 5 minutes and turn off heat. Let sit another 5 minutes. Strain off ginger and add essential oil and honey. Place in a glass bottle and refrigerate. Keeps for up to a week and a half. Do not use if you have very sensitive skin.

Love Potion Lip Balm

1 teaspoon olive oil
1 teaspoon petroleum jelly
2 teaspoons honey
1 teaspoon pure orange extract
½ teaspoon ground cinnamon

In a very small sauce pan or pot heat oil and jelly until completely liquefied. Turn off heat and add cinnamon and extract. Pour into a clean container. Apply as needed. Simply excellent! All unused portions should be kept refrigerated.

Love Potion Lip Balm II

4 Tablespoons petroleum jelly
½ teaspoon vitamin E
½ teaspoon powdered rose petals
2 drops rose essential oil
2 drops of musk fragrance oil

In a small sauce pan or pot melt vitamin E and jelly until liquefied. Next add ingredients as listed. Place in a small clean container and store in the refrigerator.

Note: If you do not have powdered rose petals at hand, you can make your own by drying fresh petals from your organic garden and placing in a coffee grinder. Pulse until pulverized. Store in a cool, dark place. Discard if it shows any signs of mold.

Galaxy Gloss

> 1 teaspoon vitamin E oil
> 2 Tablespoons petroleum jelly
> 10 drops of blue Roman chamomile essential oil
> ½ teaspoon dried chamomile flowers

Place all ingredients except essential oil into a small pot or sauce pan. Heat until jelly is melted. Let cool slightly and add essential oil. Do not strain off plant material. With this addition the gloss will turn blue, which is what we want. Place in a clean container and store in your refrigerator.

Note: Remember to do a patch test.

❧ SPECIAL REMEDIES:

Acne Poultice

> ½ Cup of dried papaya or ½ Cup fresh
> 1 Cup filtered water
> 10 drops bergamot essential oil
> ½ Cup of fresh violet flowers

In a small pot bring water to a boil, reduce heat and place papaya in along with the violet flowers. Leave on low heat for 10 minutes and then let steep covered for 1 hour. After an hour strain off plant material and papaya. Add essential oil of bergamot. Place in a clean container. To use, soak a clean cloth in solution and use as a compress on afflicted areas holding in place for 10 to 20 minutes. All unused portions should be refrigerated for no more than 4 days. This concoction is very helpful and fast acting.

Acne Salve

½ Cup of olive oil
1 Tablespoon vitamin E
1 Cup of fresh violet flowers
1 teaspoon of natural bees wax
10 drops of bergamot essential oil

In a small sauce pan or pot melt bees wax until liquefied. Place remaining items in as listed. Stir and cover for 10 minutes. Turn heat off and let mixture steep for one hour covered. After an hour remove plant material by straining and place in a clean container. Mettle or ceramic works best. Keep refrigerated. Apply to skin after cleansing. Works best on less severe cases of teen and adult acne.

Soothing Acne Bath

10 drops bergamot essential oil
10 drops lavender essential oil
½ Cup oatmeal
1 piece of cheese cloth

Combine together in a small bowl and transfer to cheese cloth. Tie into a bag and drop under hot running water. Give bag a gentle squeeze before entering. Very soothing to acne on the back and shoulders. Use up to once a week.

Natural Sunburn Treatment

10 grapes with out seeds
½ Cup cucumber chopped
2 Tablespoons aloe vera gel
½ Cup water

Mix all in a blender for a few minutes and apply to affected areas as a spot treatment. Leave on until dry and remove with cool water. Put all unused portions in the refrigerator and discard after 5 days.

Eagle Talons

4 Tablespoons vegetable oil
2 teaspoons honey
10 drops lemon essential oil

Mix all together until well incorporated. Place in a clean container and use a natural brush to apply to nails each night. This formula will help strengthen your nails which in turns helps them grow longer. Keep in the refrigerator and discard after a week.

Mehndi Henna Hand Designs

Mehndi hand designs have been done for hundreds of years by the peoples of India traditionally for wedding ceremonies. It is believed to have been started in Egypt and spread to India around the 12th century. Today this practice is still carried on and now many people are decorating their hands with natural henna just for fun. The henna is applied in various ways with the most common being with a cone. Use a piece of paper shaped into a cone with a very small hole at the end. It is similar to what cake decorators use. The henna paste is placed inside and a design is drawn onto the hand, wrist, etc. Depending on the deepness of the resulting color you would like to achieve, the paste is left on for anywhere from 3 to 12 hours or until dry. Even though the paste is a dark green or even black in color, the resulting henna tattoo is light orange to deep brown. After the henna has been left on for the time you feel comfortable with, the dried paste is washed off with water or can be scraped off dry. Underneath you have your henna mehndi. It can last for up to 4 weeks if you take care not to use hand creams or chemicals that strip the skins top layers. Keep in mind though that the henna paste is very hard to get out of clothing so don't wear anything important when doing this.

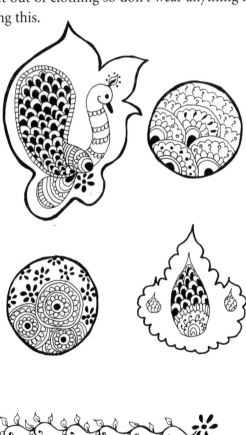

A Basic Recipe Using Henna

> 2 teaspoons dried finely ground natural henna powder
> 2 drops of eucalyptus or neroli essential oil
> Enough water to make a thick, goopy paste.

In a paper cup or metal bowl mix all ingredients well. You may have to do a bit of trial and error before getting the right paste consistency. Place into a pre-made cone and make a simple pattern on your wrist, hand, etc. Leave on as long as you like, then scrape off.

Variations:

The paint brush method:

> 2 teaspoons of natural henna powder
> 2 drops lemon essential oil
> ½ lemon cut into slices (w/ peel)
> ½ Cup water

In a small sauce pan place water and lemon. Boil for 5 minutes then reduce heat simmering for another 5 minutes. Turn heat off and let lemons sit one hour. Mix powder and essential oil together and enough lemon water to make a thin, runny paste, almost the consistency of oil paint. Using a natural fiber paint brush make designs and leave to dry. Leave on for 3 to 7 hours then rinse off with warm water.

The stencil method:

You can make a stencil out of paper by cutting out a design or buy one in a craft store. Ones depicting flowers, butterflies, hearts etc. work best and it's a good idea to keep it simple. Using the henna paste recipe, take the stencil and tape it to your hand. You can also have a friend hold it in place for you. Using the back of a spoon spread on the paste being sure to fill in all the corners of the stencil. If possible leave the stencil on until the paste sets a bit. Gently peel off stencil and leave paste on for as long as you like. Remove by scraping off or with warm water.

Note: Remember to do a patch test.

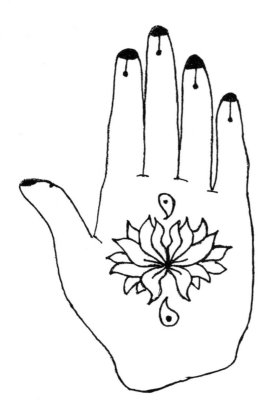

Dye Chart
~✦~✦~✦~

In the days before chemical dyes, people had to make their own by boiling plants and dunking yarn or fabric into it. You can still do this by using the plants below.

Blue: Indigo, Oregon grape.

Brown: Burdock, hops, fennel, comfrey.

Green: Sunflower leaves, sage, coltsfoot.

Orange: Sunflower, chicory.

Red: Dandelion, St. John's Wort.

Yellow: Chamomile, dandelion, fenugreek, onion skins

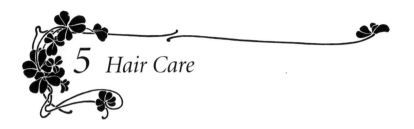

5 Hair Care

Our hair is so important to us that it deserves its own chapter and also because we do so much to it. Coloring, bleaching, straightening, harsh - unnatural hair products and heat styling all takes a major toll. Add in the effects of winter cold and the burning sun and you have a prescription for extremely damaged locks. There are many natural treatments you can use to help remedy most common hair problems. As you replace your current detergent based shampoos with organic cleansers and conditioners, you're sure to see great improvement in little or no time.

Essential Oils That Are Great for the Hair and Scalp:

Rosemary, Tea Tree, Cedarwood, Blue Roman Chamomile, Eucalyptus, Lemon, Juniper, Lavender, and YlangYlang.

Herbs That Are Great for the Hair and Scalp:

Rosemary, Sage, Chamomile, Lavender, Juniper, Arnica, Stinging Nettle, Soap Wort, Yucca and Fennel.

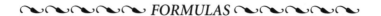 *FORMULAS*

Basic Natural Shampoo

  5 drops of lemon essential oil
  1 Cup of water
  ¼ Cup of soapwort

Place soapwort and water into a small pot. Let come to a boil than simmer for 5 minutes. Turn heat off and let stand until cool. Add essential oil. Massage into hair well and let stand for 5 minutes. Rinse out well and use a conditioner if you like.

Commercial Shampoo Additive

  10 drops of rosemary essential oil
  1 teaspoon of vanilla extract
  10 drops of chamomile essential oil

In a small bowl mix ingredients together. Add to your shampoo and shake to mix well. Be sure to shake each time before applying to hair.

Color Enhancement for Dark Hair

  5 drops of rosemary essential oil
  ¼ Cup dried sage chopped
  ½ Cup dark brewed coffee (not instant)
  1 Tablespoon of vanilla extract
  1 Cup of water

Place dried sage in a sauce pan along with water and bring to a boil. Turn heat off , cover and let steep for 2 hours. Add essential oil, pre-brewed coffee, and vanilla. Mix well. After shampooing your hair, massage mixture into hair. Let sit for 5 minutes then rinse completely. Use a conditioner if you like. Not only will your hair be deeply conditioned but shiny, manageable and more vibrant in color. Use no more than once a week.

Color Enhancement for Light/Blonde Hair

> 5 drops of lemon essential oil
> 1 Cup of dried chamomile flowers or tea
> 1 teaspoon of lemon juice
> 1 Tablespoon of banana extract
> 1 Cup of water

Bring one cup of water to a boil. Turn heat off and add chamomile, cover and let stand for 2 hours. When cool place banana extract, lemon juice and essential oil in. Mix well. After shampooing hair, work concoction into hair well. Let stand for 5 minutes in hair. Rinse well with cool water. If you have sensitive skin you may want to reduce the amount of lemon juice/essential oil. Use no more than once a week.

Rose Petal Hair Conditioner

> ½ Cup of dried rose petals or 1 Cup fresh
> 1 Cup of water
> 4 Tablespoons of mayonnaise
> 1 teaspoon of vanilla extract
> 3 drops of rose essential oil (optional)

In a sauce pan or small pot place water and rose petals. Always make sure petals are organic and free of pesticides and/or preservatives. Simmer for 5 minutes then turn the heat off. Let stand for 2 to 3 hours. When cool strain out petals and mix in mayonnaise, vanilla, and essential oil. Incorporate well. Rinse hair with water, then massage mixture into hair, especially the ends. Pile up on top of head and let stay on for 20 to

30 minutes. Covering hair with a plastic cap or wrap will help it to penetrate deep into the hair shaft. Rinse and shampoo out. Makes enough for one application.

Exotic Fruity Hair Mask

¼ avocado peeled and mashed
1 egg
½ teaspoon of vanilla extract
½ teaspoon of banana extract
5 drops of orange essential oil
2 drops of lemon essential oil

In a bowl mix all ingredients together well until completely incorporated. After rinsing hair with cool water and ringing well, smooth on mask. Pile hair on top of your head and cover with a plastic cap or wrap. Let stay on for 20 to 30 minutes. Rinse and shampoo out well. Follow up with a conditioner if you like.

Natural Hot Oil Treatment

2 Tablespoons of olive oil
2 Tablespoons of sweet almond oil
5 drops of orange essential oil
5 drops of vanilla essential oil
2 drops of lemon essential oil
½ teaspoon of honey
½ teaspoon of margarine

Place olive oil, sweet almond oil, margarine and honey in a small sauce pan. Heat until combined well. Let cool a bit and add essential oils. Mix well. Place in a clean glass container. To reheat place glass container in hot water or in a microwave for a few seconds. Best if used warm on the hair especially the ends.

Shiny Locks Conditioner

½ Cup of honey
5 drops of rosemary essential oil
½ teaspoon of olive oil

In a small bowl mix together all ingredients. Rinse hair with cool water and apply mixture to hair. Evenly distribute and work in well. Cover hair with a plastic cap or wrap and leave on for 20 to 30 minutes. Shampoo out and rinse well. Follow up with a conditioner if you like. Note: If you have dark brown to black hair keep in mind that honey is a mild lightener. You may want to substitute molasses instead.

Herbal Dandruff Help

1 Cup of Stinging Nettle dried
1 Cup of water
1 teaspoon of apple cider vinegar
2 drops lemon essential oil

Bring water and herbs to a boil. Reduce heat and let simmer for 5 minutes. Let cool and strain off plant material. Mix together with vinegar and essential oil. Massage into hair after shampooing. Rinse out well with cool water. Use as often as you like.

Hair Growth Tonic

2 Cups of apple cider vinegar
¼ Cup of peach seeds (inside of pit)
10 drops of rosemary essential oil

Boil seeds in vinegar until mixture thickens. Strain and place in a clean container. Massage into scalp for 10 minutes and shampoo out well. Keep peach seeds out of reach of children & pets as they contain cyanide.

❧ COMPLETE HAIR TREATMENT

This is a complete hair treatment from start to finish that will repair and deep condition your locks. Whether your hair is in dire need of repair or in great shape already, you will see a noticeable difference. Make sure you are able to set enough time aside for yourself to do this treatment correctly in order to obtain the best results.

Natural Hair Purifier

    1 egg
    10 drops of lemon essential oil
    ¼ Cup of water
    ¼ Cup of rum (clear/white)
    2 Tablespoons of lemon juice

In a small bowl or cup, mix all ingredients together well. You may find a blender helpful in incorporating this concoction. Note: If you have sensitive skin or dry hair you may want to cut back on the lemon additives.

Deep Conditioning Almond Hair Mask

    ¼ Cup of honey
    1 Tablespoon of almond extract
    ¼ Cup of mayonnaise
    1 teaspoon of olive oil
    2 Tablespoons of fresh fennel

In a blender place honey, finely chopped fennel and olive oil. Blend for 5 minutes or until well incorporated. Next add mayonnaise and almond extract. Blend for another 5 minutes. Keep refrigerated until ready to use.

Shine Boosting Rinse

3 Cups of water
½ Cup of dried rosemary or 1 Cup of fresh rosemary
2 Tablespoons of dried oregano
½ teaspoon of cloves

Bring water to a boil and add cloves. Turn down heat and let simmer for 5 minutes. Add herbs and let simmer for another 5 minutes. Turn heat off completely and cover. Let stand for 1 hour. Keep refrigerated until ready to use.

Step one:
Rinse hair completely with cool running water. Using the tips of your fingers massage your scalp. Ring as much of the water as you can out of your hair.

Step two:
Using the Natural Hair Purifier you prepared earlier, work it into hair. Pile hair on top of your head and leave mixture on for 5 minutes. If you rather use a commercial shampoo, follow directions of bottle.

Step three:
After the 5 minutes is up rinse hair thoroughly in cool water. Spread on the Deep Conditioning Almond Hair Mask you prepared ahead of time and work well into the ends of your hair. Cover with a plastic cap or wrap and than a warm towel. Leave on for 20 to 30 minutes.

Step four:
Rinse hair completely once again with cool water. Using the Shine Boosting Rinse or one of the other rinses in this book, pour over hair and massage in. Leave on for 5 minutes.

Step five:
Rinse hair for the last time with cool water. Air dry.

Note: People with long hair may find the need to double or even triple the recipes given. Also keep in mind that all recipes must be kept refrigerated and for no longer than a week. Always remember to do a patch test before using any of the formulas.

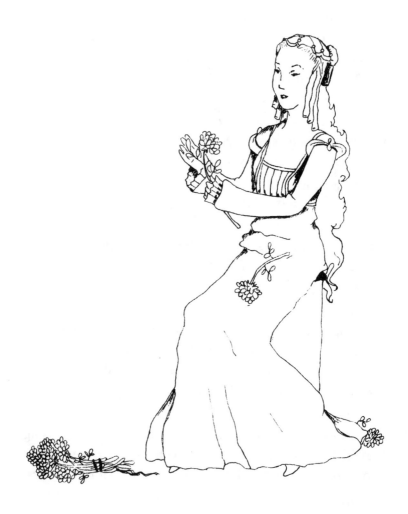

Ayurvedic Herbs & Their Ancient Uses

Vacha (Acorus calamus):
Nervine, antispasmodic, sedative, stomachache
soother, expectorant, laxative and diuretic effects.

Nagadamni (Artemisia vulgaris):
Expels worms and an expectorant.

Neem (Azadirachta indica):
Various skin disorders, antibiotic and blood disease.

Brahmi (Bacopa monnieri):
Nervous system tonic, diuretic, and sedative.

Argbhada (Cassia fistula):
Constipation, fever, and antibacterial

Devadaru (Cedrus deodara):
Fever, diarrhea, and urinary tract disorders.

Mandukaparni (Centella asiatica):
Whole body tonic, and sedative.

Jeeraka (Cuminum cyminum):
Diarrhea and dyspepsia.

Ayurvedic Herbs & Their Ancient Uses

Shati (Curcuma zedoaria):
Cough, asthma, and other respiratory problems.

Dattura (Datura metal):
Joint pain and asthma.

Garijara (Daucus carota):
Blood purifier, nervous system tonic, and jaundice.

Shankapushpi (Evolvulus alsinoides):
Anxiety, diarrhea, bronchitis, fevers,
and memory loss.

Hingu (Ferula foetida):
Cough, constipation, palpitations,
and other gastric problems.

Note: uses are based on ancient text.

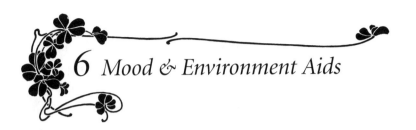

6 Mood & Environment Aids

There are many things you can do to improve your mood and well-being within your home. It need not be expensive and it need not be elaborate but the benefits will be extraordinary. The recipes below are simple, yet fun to make and leave a lot of room for experimentation.

Victorian Potpourri

3 Cups dried rose petals
½ Cup dried orange peel
2 Tablespoon of whole cloves
2 teaspoons ground nutmeg
10 drops orange essential oil

Place all ingredients in a zip lock bag and let cure for a week. Make sure to store in a cool, dark place and shake the bag every other day. When cured you can do one of two things with it. You could place it in a very pretty bowl on your coffee or side table for a light aroma or you can place potpourri in a pot of water on your kitchen stove. Keep the heat low and you can enjoy a wonderful smell throughout your house all day. If you are using the second technique, make sure it is never left unattended. Make sure you turn it off when out of the house.

࿊ CANDLES

Candles are an easy way to spread potions throughout an entire room. The following recipe is simple and inexpensive to make. Unlike artificially scented candles, you know that you are getting the full benefit of pure essential oils and nothing more. You may use the recipes for perfumes in chapter three, omitting the base oil or the simple blends below.

Candle preparation: First go to any good craft store and get a large round or square beeswax candle. If you can, try to get the natural kind and not the ones that are colored. Colored ones more than likely have more chemicals. Placing the candle on a hard, flat surface, take a Philip head screwdriver and/or long nail to poke 4 to 6 holes straight down from the top of the candle. Stop one to one-half inch from the bottom. Fill the holes with your own special oil blend, one-half inch from the top. An eyedropper works well for this application. Now light the candle and let some of the wax melt. As soon as it does, pick the candle up and roll it so the melted wax fills the holes where the oil is kept. Be very careful not to ignite the essential oils which are quite flammable. The essential oil is now trapped inside of the candle. It's best to let it sit inside of a zip lock bag for about a week to let the oils permeate the candle.

Some simple candle oil blends:

　　Romantic: Cedarwood and rose essential oil
　　Love potion: Jasmine essential oil and musk fragrance oil
　　Refreshing: Orange and Narcissus essential oil
　　Spicy: Bergamot and patchouli essential oil

Mix as much or as little as you like to get the exact fragrance you're looking for. The amount of oil you will need all depends on the size of the candle you will be working with.

Variations:

Victorian Flower Candles

> A few cured homemade Aromatherapy candles
> Some dried pot pourrie or flowers
> Some dried leaves and orange peel

You can use the candle blends above or scent them with a blend ratio of 1 part vanilla and 1part jasmine essential oil. Prepare as above. Using a knife or nail to score the candle, make a line ½ to 1 inch from the bottom of the candle. This will serve as your guide. Using glue, spread onto the candle under the line you made. A paint brush works best. Wait a few seconds for the glue to set a bit and then begin to attach flowers, leaves, peel etc. When done, place candles on a hard surface in a dry place to let glue set completely. Overnight it best. Once dry, store candles in a cool, dark place.

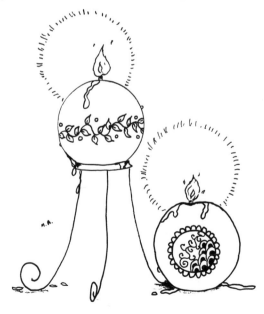

Mehndi Candles

    A few cured homemade Aromatherapy candles
    Dried ground cinnamon
    Black non-toxic craft paint - paint brush
    or
    A black thin tip permanent marker

Use the candle blends above or this special combination, 1 part orange and 1 part sandalwood essential oil. Prepare as above. Taking a cured candle, score a line around the bottom half. This will become your guide for keeping the mehndi design in the right place and later the ground cinnamon. Using the paint or marker method, draw a mehndi design all around the candle or a medallion in one spot. Let the candle sit and dry for 1 or 2 hours. When dry to the touch it is ready for the next step, addition of the ground cinnamon. In a small bowl or paper plate sprinkle on enough cinnamon for your candle to be rolled in. Spread on glue to the bottom half of the candle and let set a few seconds. Place candle in cinnamon and roll until all areas are covered well. Place on a hard dry surface overnight. Store in a cool, dry place.

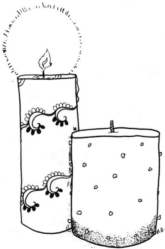

❧ DREAM PILLOWS

These little pillows can be made quite quickly and used to help induce sleep, scent clothes and more. Once you start, it hard to stop making them for yourself and loved ones!

2 squares of cotton fabric

Stuffing (organic cotton works best but use whatever is on hand)

Dried rose petals and/or orange zest powdered

Lavender essential oil

Lily of the valley fragrance oil

I haven't given the exact amounts as you may want to make different size pillows. It all depends on the materials you have on hand. Using a zip-lock bag, place the stuffing inside, along with the petals and or zest (peel) making sure to well incorporate everything. Use about 10 drops of each oil for a very small pillow (5 ½ x 4) or 20 drops of each for a larger pillow. You may have to experiment to see how much you'll ultimately need. Let the stuffing sit for a week inside the bag. For the pillow casing, place right sides together. Sew all sides but leave a small opening in the middle of one side so you will be able to turn the pillow inside out through it. Turn pillow case inside out and stuff through small whole left not sewed. Pack well and sew closed. Very calming when placed inside of your bed pillow case. Please keep in mind that this type of pillow should never be washed. If the scent is no longer evident you can either reopen it and add more essential oils or make a brand new one. The color you make your pillow can be almost as important as what you place inside. According to ancient Tibetan beliefs, colors have a power to change out moods and cares. Colors like blue, turquoise, and green help induce relaxation, balance, dreaming etc. so they would be the perfect color for your pillows.

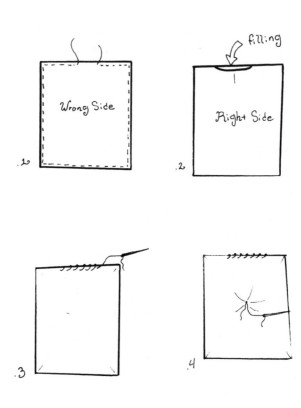

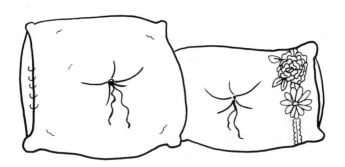

❧ ROOM MISTS

This is a great alternative to the commercial room deodorizers and fresheners. Try this basic recipe for use all over your house or the more specific variations.

1 Cup water
20 drops lavender essential oil
¼ teaspoon honey

In a spray bottle combine all ingredients. Shake bottle well before use. Store in refrigerator in between use.

Variations:

Bedroom Mist

1 Cup water
10 drops rose essential oil
10 drops sandalwood essential oil
2 or 3 drops musk fragrance oil (optional)
¼ teaspoon honey

Prepare as above.

Kitchen Mist

1 Cup water
20 drops tea tree essential oil
5 drops lavender essential oil
¼ teaspoon honey

Prepare as above

Bathroom Mist

1 Cup water
10 drops bergamot essential oil
10 drops lemon essential oil
¼ teaspoon honey

Prepare as above

&. LOVE SACHETS

> 2 square or rectangle pieces of fabric or 4 squares of lace
> Dried rose petals
> Dried clover blossoms
> Rose essential oil
> Musk fragrance oil
> Ground cinnamon

Place enough rose petals and clover blossoms to fill your desired pillow size into a zip-lock bag. Add oils. Let sit in a dark, cool place for 3 days. Sew three sides of your pillow up and fill with stuffing. Sew remaining side closed or place buttons on the edge so you can reopen to refill with new material. You can make very pretty sachets by simply sewing lace on as you would for putting a bow on a present and/or silk flowers representing what is inside. They make excellent gifts which recipients will treasure, long after the scent is gone. They can be used to scent clothes and bedding as well.

&. LETTERS WITH REAL MEANING

Whether you are sending a get well card to a friend or a long letter, you can make it mean so much more by adding essential oils. You can make a blend that will scent all of your stationery or choose a special aroma for the occasion.

Some simple blends:

> **Uplifting blend:** Lavender and bergamot essential oil
> **Aphrodisiac blend:** Sandalwood and jasmine essential oil
> **Cheering blend:** Ylang ylang and orange essential oil

Using a few cotton balls, soak in essential oil or blends of your choice. Place stationary inside of a zip-lock bag. Lay on a flat surface and add cotton balls. Try to separate the paper from the cotton balls as the essential oil may stain it. Let sit for 1 to 2 weeks before using.

❧ HOMEMADE INCENSE

I have found that there are many ways of making incense with the most common being loose, cylinder, stick or cone. I will be showing you how to make the essayist sorts, loose non-combustible and incense blocks. If you were to make the combustible cone, stick etc. type of incense the main ingredients would be:

A base wood which has been pulverized such as cedar, sandalwood etc.

An aromatic substance such as fragrance oils or loose incense

An igniting substance such as saltpeter

A glue to hold everything together such as tragacanth

Lastly a liquid which could be olive oil, flower waters, wine etc.

You would mix everything together and weigh it. This is because you would need to do a little math to see what would be 10% of the total weight as this would equal the amount of igniter you would need to add. The glue would be added last and then you would start forming the mixture into a cone shape. They then will take around 1 to 2 weeks to cure and dry completely. In the mean time you have to turn them each day to assure they don't crack. I find it all rather tedious, hence, why I have provided these easier to make recipes that come out just as pleasing.

Combustible Amour Incense

> 2 Tablespoons powdered orris root
> ½ teaspoon powdered sugar
> ¼ teaspoon ground cinnamon
> 5 drops rose essential oil
> 1 or 2 drops olive oil

Grind each ingredient separately in a coffee grinder or by hand with a mortar and pestle.

In a small bowl, mix dry ingredients together well. Add oils. Combine to make a paste, you may find the need to add 1-2 drops of water. Shape into little square cubes, long blocks or pea sized balls. Cure in your oven for 5-10 minutes on very low heat, or let bake in the sun. Keep in a tin until ready to use. Dried rose petals, benzoin gum and or pine needles can also be added for extra scent.

Non-Combustible Loose Incense

First, before you prepare the loose incense mixture you will need to purchase little charcoal disks which can be found in most health food stores. The incense you make is placed on top of the lighted charcoal which burns and heats the incense. This makes things much simpler and allows for more creativity.

In a coffee grinder you can combine the following ingredients:

> Dried rose petals
> Ground cinnamon
> Pine needles
> Clover blossoms
> Dried ground orris root

Pulverize to a fine powder. Add essential oils and let mixture cure in a tin or glass container with a tight fitting lid. This can take up to 1 ½ to 2 weeks. The key is to make a fine powder and keep it as dry and loose as possible. Once it is cured, it is ready to use. A great way of starting the charcoal going is to take it and place it over your stoves burner. Using barbecue tongs, turn it over and over until a thin layer of ash forms. Place on a incense burner and sprinkle incense over the coal.

Another extremely easy way of making your own incense is to buy unscented incense sticks or cones. These are primed with the igniter, base wood, glue, etc. but with no scent. You add the aroma yourself by letting it soak in fragrance oil, essential oils or coat with loose incense powder.
Please keep in mind though that you should never leave incense where a child may have access to it. Never leave it burning unattended and always use an incense burner made of clay, stone, brass, etc.

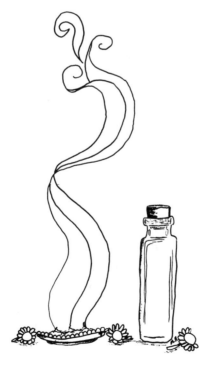

❧ HOMEMADE TEAS AND ELIXIRS

Most teas are made in the same way, either by infusion or decoction. The infusion method is for tender parts of a plant such as the flowers, leaves, fruit etc. You would go about this by placing herbs in a container and pouring just boiling water over them and letting it steep for 5 to 10 minutes. A decoction on the other hand it for tougher parts of a plant such as the root, stem & bark. For this method you would place all the plant matter in a pot of water and bring it to a boil. You would then turn heat down and let it simmer for up to one hour. Keep in mind that one third of the water will probably evaporate, so you'll need to add extra to compensate. Elixirs can be made in a number of ways such as a cold infusion, syrup, tincture, etc. Here are a few delectable teas and helpful elixirs you will want to try for yourself.

Soothing Almond Tea

3 black tea bags (a mixture of black tea and orange pekoe works well also)
2 Cups of boiling water
4 Cups water
½ Cup sugar (or use honey to taste)
5 Tablespoons fresh lemon juice
2 teaspoons pure almond extract
½ teaspoon pure vanilla extract
¼ Cup slivered almonds

Combine tea bags and 2 cups of water in a small sauce pan. Bring to a boil, turn heat off and let steep 30 minutes. In another pot mix 4 cups of water with sugar and rest of ingredients except for slivered almonds. Bring to a simmer and turn heat off. Remove tea bags and pour tea into other mixture. Reheat, add slivered almonds and serve.

Dandelion Tea

> 1 Cup of dandelion flowers, carefully washed
> 4 Cups water
> 1 teaspoon orange zest

Bring water to a rolling boil. Place flowers and zest in another pot and pour boiling water over them. This is a classic infusion. Cover and let stand 15 minutes. Strain off all plant material and sweeten as desired. Traditionally used as a liver purifier and treatment for anemia. Be mindful that dandelion is a diuretic.

Love Potion Tea

> 1 Cup fresh lovage leaves, flowers, or root or ½ Cup dried
> 3 Cups water
> Honey to taste

Bring water to a boil and use either the decoction method for the root or the infusion technique for the lovage (Levisticum offcinale) leaves, flowers etc. Used for thousands of years by many nomadic peoples as an aphrodisiac and soother.

Note: people with kidney problems and who are pregnant should not ingest this tea.

Royal Russian Tea Blend

> The contents of 6 black tea bags
> ½ teaspoon lemon zest
> ½ teaspoon orange zest
> ½ teaspoon ground cloves

½ Cup sugar or honey to taste

In a coffee grinder or by using a mortar and pestle, grind all ingredients together until well incorporated. Store in a tin container with a tight fitting lid. Place one teaspoon in a tea ball and drop into boiling water. Let steep and serve.

Rose Hip Tea

½ Cup dried rose hips

¼ teaspoon orange zest

Place both ingredients in a coffee grinder or mortar and pestle. Grind well. Store in a tin container with a tight fitting lid. Use 3 teaspoons in a tea ball and lower into boiling water. Let steep 10 minutes and reheat if necessary. Known to contain a high amount of vitamin C, rose hips have been traditionally used to strengthen the heart and calm the stomach.

Note: some hybrid roses do not produce rose hips. Rosa laevigata and Rosa canina species produce edible rose hips. Always make sure plants are organically grown as well.

Violet Sleep Elixir

1 Cup of fresh violet flowers

2 Cups water

¾ Cup of honey

Place flowers into boiling water. Turn off heat and let stand 24 hours covered in the refrigerator. Strain and add mixture to another 1 cup of water, bring to a rapid boil and then reduce heat. Simmer until liquid is reduced by half. Use ¼ cup at a time.

Sleep Syrup

1 Cup fresh Chamomile leaves or ½ Cup dried

1 Cup water
½ Cup honey

In a small sauce pan bring water to a boil. Add fresh chamomile and simmer 5 minutes. Turn heat off and let stand 30 minutes. In another sauce pan heat honey. When warm add ½ cup of chamomile tea being sure to stir well. Let cool. Store in a glass bottle with a cork. Bottles with tight fitting lids may burst. Always store in the refrigerator. Use 1 teaspoon at a time.

Note: not to be used by infant due to the honey component.

Spirit Lifter

½ Cup chopped fresh rosemary
1 16 oz. bottle of sweet white wine

Place chopped herb in white wine bottle and let steep for 1 week in the refrigerator. Take one tablespoon at a time. Used traditionally to lift the spirits and chase away depression. Note: Not to be given to children or ingested by people with epilepsy or high blood pressure.

Variation:

Rosemary Tincture

½ Cup fresh rosemary or ¼ Cup dried
2 ½ Cups vodka or rum

Place in a glass container with a lid. Let stand in your refrigerator for ½ to 2 weeks. Strain off plant material and store in the refrigerator. Use ½ teaspoon at a time. This tincture can also be used on cuts as a disinfectant.

Note: Not to be given to children or ingested by people with epilepsy or high blood pressure.

Chinese Herbs & Their Ancient Uses

∽∼∽∼∽∼∽∼∽∼∽∼∽∼∽∼

Agrimony (Xianhecao Agrimonia eupatoria):
Internal bleeding and stomach ulcers.

Wild Ginger (or sheng jiang Asarum canadense):
Headaches, nausea, and colds.

Gentain (or long dan cao Gentiana lutea):
Various skin conditions, bladder infections,
and rheumatic pain.

Licorice (or gan cao Glycyrrhiza spp.):
Gastric problems, detoxification, and coughs.

Dandelion (or pu gong ying
Tarazacum mongolicum):
Liver cleanser, whole body tonic, and diuretic.

Green Tea (Camellia sinensis):
Aid in digestion, skin conditioned, and tonic.

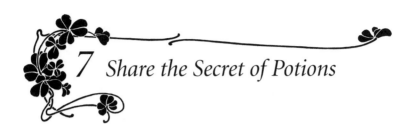

7 Share the Secret of Potions

Now that you have learned how to prepare all sorts of pleasing potions for yourself, why not share the experience with others? A gift that is homemade with love is undoubtedly the best kind. Below you will find recipes that are easy, inexpensive, and sure to be treasured by the recipients plus some wrapping ideas.

❧ GIFTS FOR HER

Here are a few formulas that any women would enjoy receiving and using. Don't feel bad if you can't help but try them out on yourself first.

Pixie Dust

½ Cup arrowroot powder
½ Cup cornstarch
1 teaspoon ground dried orange zest
15 drops neroli essential oils
1 drop of red food coloring

Blend all together in a blender until well incorporated. Place in a clean container such as a large salt shaker. Use as a lightly scented dusting powder or can be sprinkled on bed sheets. Refrigerate all unused portions.

Variations:

Queen of Love

½ Cup cornstarch
½ Cup arrowroot powder
½ teaspoon ground cinnamon
15 drops rose essential oil
2 or 3 drops red food coloring

Prepare as above.

Queen of the Night

½ Cup cornstarch
½ Cup arrowroot powder
2 Tablespoons orris root powder
15 drops jasmine essential oil
1 drop purple food coloring

Prepare as above.

Homemade Body Soaps

Most homemade soap recipes call for lye crystals. Due to this caustic ingredient, the formula must be handled very cautiously and all components must be combined carefully. The recipes below are extra simple to make as they use natural, unscented pre-made soap.

Flower Petal Glycerin Soap

1 bar natural unscented glycerin soap
½ Cup ground dried rose petals, lavender, pot marigold, chamomile, honeysuckle, violet, and/or clover.
½ teaspoon pure vanilla extract or 5 drops essential oil
2 to 3 Cups water
An empty tea box

Line the inside of an empty tea bag box with aluminum foil and set aside. In a small sauce pan bring water to a boil. Turn heat off. Using the soaps plastic wrapper or a zip lock bag with the whole soap inside, dunk in water until liquefied. Lift bag with tongs as it is quite hot. Make sure you dry off any water that may be on the outside of your bag. With scissors cut off one of the corners of the bag. This will allow you to pour the melted soap into the tea box mold. After pouring soap into the tea box, add vanilla and then dried flower petals of choice. Mix in with a spoon and smooth out top so that it is even and flat. Let soap cool for 2 to 3 hours. Once cool, use a knife to cut 3 bars. Wrap in tissue paper and let cure 1 week. After it has cured it is ready to use. If you want to get a little more fancy, you can purchase shaped soap molds. I've found that ones made of plastic are best as they bend and flex making it easier to remove finished soaps.

Variations:

Oatmeal Almond Soap

> 1 bar natural, unscented glycerin soap
> ¼ Cup ground oatmeal
> 2 Tablespoons ground almonds
> 5 drops chamomile essential oil
> Prepare as above.
> Orange Cinnamon Morning Soap
> 1 bar natural, unscented glycerin soap
> 4 Tablespoons chopped orange zest
> ¼ teaspoon ground cinnamon

> Prepare as above.

Herbal Body Soap

Here is another way of making delightful homemade soap easily. Look for pre-made soap that is unscented and as natural as possible.

½ unscented white beauty bar
¼ Cup dried chamomile, strawberry leaves, clover, lavender, or stinging nettle.
5 drops chamomile essential oil

In a double boiler place grated soap and heat until smooth. The soap will not melt to the consistency of the liquefied glycerin soap, but will instead become a thick paste. Remove from heat and add herbs and essential oil of choice. Mix with a wooden spoon until well incorporated. Remove from pot and smooth well into an aluminum foil lined tea box. Let cool completely for 4 to 6 hours. When cooled, slice into 3 bars. Wrap tightly in a couple of layers of tissue paper and let cure for 2 weeks in a dry, dark place. With this sort of soap, the longer it is allowed to cure, the better it becomes.

Spicy Hard Perfume

2 Tablespoons jojoba or sweet almond oil
6 drops bergamot essential oil
10 drops jasmine essential oil
6 drops petit grain essential oil or fragrance oil
½ teaspoon natural bees wax

In a sauce pan melt oil and bees wax together. Pour into a clean container and refrigerate. Dab on anytime you want a hint of natural scent.

Variations:

Victorian Vanilla

2 Tablespoons jojoba or sweet almond oil
¼ teaspoon crushed, dried rose petals (optional)
2 drops rose essential oil
5 drops vanilla essential oil
½ teaspoon natural bees wax

Prepare as above.

Mandarin Dreams

2 Tablespoons jojoba or sweet almond oil
5 drops mandarin orange essential oil
5 drops ylang ylang essential oil
¼ teaspoon ground cloves
½ teaspoon bees wax

Prepare as above.

❧ GIFTS FOR HIM

Here are secret potions guaranteed to bring the fire of romance back into his heart! Scientists who study the effect of scents on the human libido have isolated specific scents that have been shown to clinically increase arousal in men. Here are a few excellent concoctions to try using the results of this latest research.

Oriental Five Spice Soap

1 bar natural, unscented glycerin soap
2 Tablespoons Chinese Five Spice seasoning
2 drops lemon essential oil (optional)
2 to 4 Cups water
An empty tea box

Line an empty tea box with aluminum foil and set aside. Cut glycerin soap into cubes. Place soap and seasoning into a zip-lock bag. In a small sauce pan bring water to a boil. Turn heat off and dunk bag containing soap into water until melted. Remove with tongs. Be sure to dry off the outside of the bag completely. Holding the bag over the tea box which will serve as your mold, cut off one of the corners. Pour in. Let cool for 2 to 3 hours. Once completely cool, cut into 3 bars. Wrap in tissue paper and let cure 1 week.

Mint Foot Soak

    1 Cup fresh mint leaves or ½ Cup dried
    ½ Cup dried comfrey
    ¼ Cup brown rice
    Cheese cloth

Mix ingredients together and divide in 2. Place in the center of a square of cheese cloth. Bring corners together and secure with a piece of string. To use, pour very hot water into a large bowl or foot bath. Add bath bag and let water cool to a comfortable temperature. Helps to soothe tired feet and relieve swelling. Keep unused portions in the refrigerator.

Love Potion Massage Oil for Men

    ½ Cup jojoba or sweet almond oil
    2 Tablespoons olive oil
    ¼ Cup uncooked pumpkin flesh
    ½ teaspoon ground cinnamon
    ¼ teaspoon ground nutmeg
    ⅛ teaspoon ginger
    ½ teaspoon allspice

Cut pumpkin into cubes and place into a blender. Pulse a

couple of times and add rest of ingredients. Blend on high until completely liquefied and incorporated. Pour into a glass container with a lid and store in the refrigerator.

Aromatic Fire Place Logs

2 Tablespoons orris root powder
½ Cup fresh pine needles
1 teaspoon benzoin essential oil/gum
5 drops pine essential oil
1 Tablespoon water
A few pieces of brown paper

In a blender, mix all ingredients well. It should be a thick paste. Take a small rectangle of brown paper (grocery bags work well) about 5 inches by 11 inches and lay flat on a hard surface. At one end make a line of pine filling and start tightly rolling the paper. Once rolled, secure it with a couple pieces of string. Using your fingers, dip them in water and spread over seem. Let logs cure in a cool, dark place for 1 week. Place a few on a roaring fire for a real treat.

❧ GIFTS FOR CHILDREN

Not only will children be very appreciative to receive the gift ideas below but will love to help you make them as well.

Mint Lollipops

½ Cup fresh mint or ¼ Cup dried
1 ¼ Cup white granulated sugar
2 Cups light corn syrup
A few drops green food coloring
5 drops peppermint flavoring (optional)
12 wooden sticks

Cover a cookie sheet with parchment paper that has been lightly buttered or sprayed with cooking spray. Set aside. In a double boiler combine sugar, corn syrup, mint leaves and food coloring. Cook over low heat for about 5 minutes or until sugar dissolves. Cover and cook over low heat about 8 minutes more. Insert a candy thermometer to determine when it reaches a temperature of 300 degrees which would mean it is at hard crack stage. Stir in flavoring and remove from heat. Quickly pour through a strainer into another pot to remove plant material. Set aside to thicken a bit. Arrange wooden sticks 6 inches apart on a cookie sheet. Drop hot candy from a tablespoon over sticks to make a 2 to 3 inch circles or squares. Let cool in the refrigerator. Wrap in plastic wrap. Mint is known to help calm the nerves, soothe the stomach and aid in digestion.

Note: Not to be given to infants.

Candied Orange Peel

6 large organic oranges
½ Tablespoon salt
2 Cups white granulated sugar
a few drops of yellow food coloring (optional)

Cut peel off of all the oranges. Try to remove as much of the white membrane as possible. Fill a sauce pan with 5 cups of water and add salt and peels. Using a plate, place over peels in water to be sure they all stay to the bottom of the pot. Let stand overnight in the refrigerator. Drain off water and rinse well in a colander. In a pot, cover peels with cold water and heat until it comes to a boil. Drain off water. Do this step three times. Using a knife or kitchen scissors, cut peel into strips. In a pot mix together sugar, peel, food coloring and ½ cup of orange juice. Heat and stir until sugar dissolves completely.

Continue to cook over low heat until peels become soft and translucent. Drain off liquid and roll peels in a dish of white granulated sugar. Place on a metal drying rack to cool. Store in a container with a lid in the refrigerator. The peel of the orange has been traditionally used in Chinese medicine for help with digestion and as an energy booster.

Note: Only use organically grown fruit.

Banana Bubble Bath

½ bar of unscented, natural glycerin soap
2 Tablespoons pure banana extract
¼ Cup water
5 drops coconut fragrance oil (optional)
¼ Cup yucca extract

In a sauce pan bring water to a boil. Turn heat off and dunk a zip-lock bag containing soap in water. Do this until it melts completely. Remove with tongs and dry the outside of the bag off. In a glass container pour liquefied soap, extract and water. Cap, bottle and shake well. Shake before each use.

Calming Hard Perfume for Children

¼ Cup sweet almond or jojoba oil
2 Tablespoons olive oil
½ teaspoon honey
2 Tablespoons dried lavender (optional)
10 drops lavender essential oil
5 drops geranium essential oil
1 Tablespoon natural bees wax

In a small pot or sauce pan, melt together all ingredients. Stir constantly. Place in a clean container with a lid and let cool in the refrigerator. Store in the refrigerator to extend it's shelf life. Children will love to have their own natural perfume. The hidden quality of this aromatic blend is that it will help children to calm down and get ready for bed.

❧ GIFTS FOR ALL

The following recipes can be made and given to any loved one including yourself.

Healing Salve

¼ Cup petroleum jelly
1 Tablespoon olive oil
1 teaspoon liquid lanolin (optional)
½ Cup dried lavender
¼ Cup dried or fresh strawberry leaves

In a sauce pan over low heat melt jelly and olive oil until liquefied. Add herbs and turn heat down very low. Cook for up to 1 hour or until herbs look crispy. Remove from heat and strain off plant material. Quickly add lanolin, stir and pour into a small clean glass container. Store in the refrigerator. Strawberry leaves have been used for centuries to help heal a variety of skin conditions and eruptions.

Aromatic Stones

Stone recipe:

2 Cups all purpose white flour
1 Cup water
1 Cup table salt
1 teaspoon white glue
2 to 4 drops food coloring of choice

In a large mixing bowl combine all ingredients and mix

well with a wooden spoon. Sprinkle a little flour on a hard flat surface and turn dough out onto it. Kneed a few times and divide into tablespoon sized amounts. Using your hands, roll and mold into stone shapes. Place stones on a cookie sheet and bake at 300 degrees for about 1 hour. Remove and let cool on a cookie rack for 1 hour. Move to a container with a lid and let cure 1 week.

Aromatic stone blends:

You can do one of two things to scent your stones. You can scent stones individually with each oil or you can make a blend of oils and scent all the stones. You can use aromatherapy or fragrance oils but keep in mind that the latter does not have any medicinal properties, just aroma.

Love: Rose, Musk, and Cinnamon
Tropics Call: Peach, Coconut and Mango
Night Queen: Jasmine and Strawberry
Whispers: Cherry, Vanilla, and Almond
White Flowers: Lily of the Valley and Sandalwood

In a plastic bag, drop a handful of stones. Add oils and let soak in for 5 days. The stones are porous so they will draw the oils inside and keep the scent for a long time. Once your stones have cured, place them on a small ceramic/pottery plate. Tea cups, sea shells or miniature flower pots work nicely as well. Position them on your coffee or kitchen table. Just like potpourri the stones will give off a pleasant light aroma for a time and can be re-scented quite easily by refreshing with the oils.

Friendship Tea

½ Cup dried apple

½ teaspoon cinnamon

½ Cup fresh honeysuckle flowers or ¼ Cup dried

Combine all ingredients well. You can either divide it into separate portions which would be about 2 tablespoons or brew a whole pot. For the latter, bring water to a boil in a tea pot. Place tea in another pot with a pourable spout. Pour boiling water over tea and steep for about 10 minutes. Place a strainer over the cup and pour each portion. Store all unused potions in the refrigerator.

❧ GIFT PRESENTATION

Just as there are many gifts to make and present to loved ones, there are many creative ways of wrapping, packing and bestowing your gift. Be sure to try some of the ideas below.

Wrapping it:

- Use a square of fabric such as: Cotton, satin, velvet or even lace. Bring the corners together and tie with a ribbon or piece of string.
- Try taking some natural brown paper that is large enough to wrap your gift. After you have done so, glue potpourri or dried flowers to the outside for an interesting and fragrant effect.
- Find a nice natural basket and fill it with either fine hay, shredded paper or potpourri. Place your gift(s) inside and cover with cellophane or tulle. This works great for aromatic candles, elixirs in glass bottles and bath gifts.

Add ons:

- Take a bouquet of dried flowers and affix them to the outside of your gift. You can use the secret flower meaning chart to find the perfect ones.

• Sea shells make the perfect accompaniment to bath items such as salts, crystals, etc. They look wonderful on the outside of the gift but can also be used later as a ladle for the salts and a holder for aromatic stones.

• Make or buy a plain gift card and glue potpourri, dried flowers or simply scent with your favorite essential oil. Write a personal message and tie it to the gift.

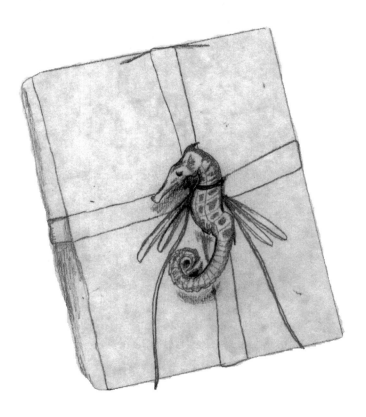

The Tibetan Thought About Colors

People of different parts of Asia have long thought that colors that surround us hold the power to control our moods and feelings. Now scientists are finding that there is a good amount of truth to these ancient beliefs and are studying into them further. Here are a few examples the conditions that can be helped through the Tibetan belief of the healing power of colors.

Purple: Alleviates panic, paranoia, and mental strain.

Blue: Eases stress, mind block, and panic.

Orange: Addresses mental tiredness and depression.

Green: Quells lack of security and trauma.

It was thought that in order to heal ones self, the person can either be surrounded with the specific color or visualize the hue for 10 minutes through meditation

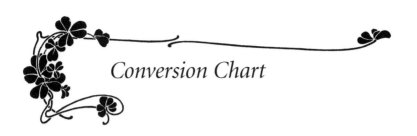

Conversion Chart

Essential / Fragrance Oils:

25 Drops = ¼ teaspoon
50 Drops = ½ teaspoon
75 Drops = ¾ teaspoon = ⅛ ounce
150 Drops = 1 ½ teaspoon = ¼ ounce

Dry

¼ Cup = 4 Tablespoons = 2 ounces
1 Cup = 16 Tablespoons = 8 ounces
2 Cups = 1 pint
4 Cups = 1 quart

Wet

¼ Cup = 2 fluid ounces = 60 ml
1 Cup = 8 fluid ounces = 250 ml

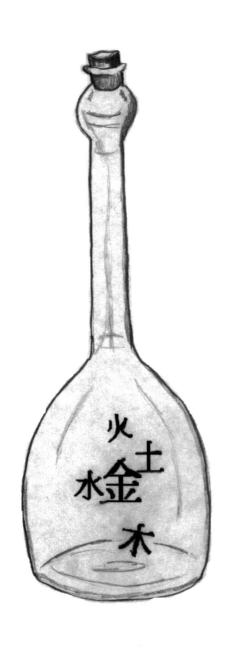

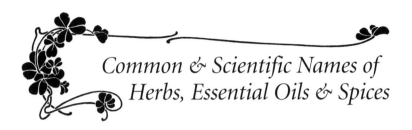

Common & Scientific Names of Herbs, Essential Oils & Spices

ALLSPICE: Lindera benzoin Also known as Jamaica Pepper

ALOE VERA: Aloe spp. Also known as Zanzibar aloe, Curaiao, and Barbados.

ANISE: Pimpinella anisum Also known as Sweet Cumin

APPLE: Pyrus malus

ARNICA: Arnica montana Also known as Wolf's and Leopard's Bane

ARROWROOT: M. arundinacea Also known as Purple Arrowroot and Brazilian Arrowroot.

AVOCADO: genus Persea

BASIL: Ocimum basilicum Also known as St. Josephwort and Sweet Basil.

BEE BALM: Milissa officinalis Also known as Melissa, Lemon Balm, Honey Plant, and Sweet Balm.

BERGAMOT: Citrus bergamia Also known as Bergamia.

BLACKBERRY: Rubus species Also known as Dewberry and Bramble.

BLUEBERRY: Vaccinium corybosum Also known as Swamp Blueberry and Highbush Blueberry.

BLACK MULBERRY: Morus nigra Also known as White Mulberry, Red Mulberry and Texas Mulberry.

BURDOCK: Articum lappa Also known as Burr.

CALENDULA: Calendula officinalis Also known as Marigold, Pot Marigold, and Hollygold.

CARDAMOM: Elettaria cardamomum

CARROT: Daucus carota

CATNIP: Nepeta cataria Also known as Catmint, Field Balm and Catswort.

CHAMOMILE: Chamaemelum nobile (Roman) & Matricaria recutita (German) Also known as (Roman) Garden Chamomile, English Chamomile, and True Chamomile. (German) Blue Chamomile, Hungarian Chamomile.

CHERRY: (demestacated) Prunus (wild) Prunus virginiana Also known as Wild Black Cherry and Choke Cherry.

CINNAMON: Cinnamomum zeylanicum Also known as Madagascar Cinnamon, Ceylon Cinnamon, and Cinnamon Bark.

CLARY SAGE: Salvia sclarea Also known as Clary Wort, Eye Bright and See Bright.

CLOVES: Engenia aromatica Also known as Caryophyllus.

CLOVER: Trifolium pratense Also known as Purple Clover, Sweet Clover and Trufolium.

COMFREY: Symphytum officinale Also known as Knitbone, Healing Herb, and Boneset.

CORIANDER: Coriandrum sativum Also known as Chinese Parsley.

CUCUMBER: Cucumis sativus

CUMIN: Cuminum cyminum Also known as Roman Caraway.

DANDELION: Taraxacum officinale Also known as Wild Endive and Lion's Tooth.

ECHINACEA: Echinacea angustifolia Also known as Purple Cone Flower.

EUCALYPTUS: Eucalyptus globulus Also known as Lemon Scented Eucalyptus, Australian Fever Tree, and Scented Gum Tree.

FENNEL: Foeniculum vulgare Also known as Carosella and Finocchio.

GERANIUM: Geranium maculatum Also known as Pelargonium and Rose Geranium.

GINGER: Zingiber officinale Also known as Jamaican Ginger and Cochin Ginger.

GOLDENSEAL: Hydrastis canadensis Also known as Yellow Root, Indian Paint, Indian Turmeric, and Yellow Puccoon.

HONEYSUCKLE: Diervilla lonicera Also known as Japanese Honeysuckle.

IRISH MOSS: Chondrus crispus

LAVENDER: Lavandula angustifolia Also known as Common Lavender and English Lavender.

LEMON: Citrus limon

LETTUCE: Lactuca sativa

MARJORAM: Origanum majorana Also known as Sweet Marjoram and Knotted Marjoram.

MINT: Mentha spp. Also known as Peppermint, Spearmint, etc.

MUSTARD: Brassica nigra Also known as Black Mustard.

NEW JERSEY TEA: Ceanot americanus

NUTMEG: Myristica fragrans Also known as Nutmeg Apple.

ORANGE FLOWER: Citrus aurantium var. amara Also known as:Neroli and Orange Blossom.

OREGANO: Origanum vulgare Also known as Wild Marjoram, Grove Marjoram and Common Oregano.

ORRIS ROOT: Florentine iris Also known as Iris.

PAPAYA: Carica papaya Also known as Pawpaw.

PARSLEY: Petroselinum crispum Also known as Rock Selinon.

PATCHOULI: Pogostemon cablin Also known as Puchaput.

PINEAPPLE: Ananas comosus

RASPBERRY: Rubus idaeus Also known as Hindberry.

ROSE: Rosa spp. Also known as Wild Rose, Cabbage Rose, Provence Rose, and Damask.

ROSEHIPS: Rosa canina Also known as Hipberry.

ROSEMARY: Rosmarinus officinalis Also known as Incensier and Rosemarine.

SANDALWOOD: Santalum album Also known as Sanders Wood and Indian Sandalwood.

SAGE: Salvia officinalis Also known as Spanish Sage and True Sage.

SOAPWORT: Saponaria officinalis Also known as Bouncing Bet.

STAR ANISE: Illicium verum Also known as Chinese Anise and Illicium.

STRAWBERRY: (domesticated) Fragaria vesca (wild) Fragaria virginiana

TEA TREE: Melaleuca alternifolia Also known as Ti-Tree, Melasol, and Ti-Trol.

TURMERIC: Curcuma longa Also known as Curcuma.

VANILLA: Vanilla planifolia Also known as Mexican Vanilla and Common Vanilla.

VIOLET: Viola odorata Also known as English Violet, Blue Violet and Garden Violet.

YUCCA ROOT: Yucca filamentose Also known as Cassava and Soapweed.

YLANG YLANG: Cananga ordorata

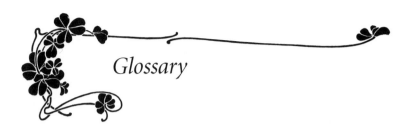

Glossary

ACNE: Prunus amygdalus A skin condition where the pours get repeatedly clogged causing pustules and inflammation. Can lead to scaring in severe cases.

ALMOND: Nut related to the peach which when used ground up helps to exfoliate and sluff off old skin sells. May also be used in pure extract form to soothe the skin and add a pleasant aroma to the finished concoction.

ANTI-INFLAMMATORY: An element that reduces swelling of the skin and helps with tenderness.

Antiseptic: An element that halts the growth of bacteria and micro-organisms.

APPLE: Pyrus malus A fruit that contains malic acid which acts as an antioxidant. Very useful for use in skin preparations especially to calm irritations. Do not use seeds as they contain toxins.

AROMATIC: A pleasing aroma that also holds the power to heal. Examples are pure essential oils and blends.

Aromatherapy: The art of using essential oils for healing and aromatic pleasure.

AYURVEDA: or ayurvedic medicine. Ayur meaning life and veda meaning knowledge it is the ancient practice of holistic medicine in India.

BAKING SODA: Also known as bicarbonate of soda. Can be used in hundreds of ways such as for natural deodorizing and cleansing.

BOTANICAL: Having to do with the healing properties in plants.

CANOLA OIL: Also known as rapeseed oil. Can be found in most food stores and is used as a base oil and additive to natural formulas for the skin.

DECOCTION: The process of boiling tough plant material such as barks and roots in water to obtain the healing properties. Can be used then in teas, poultices, masks etc.

EGG: Used in masks and hair treatments to hold things together. Helps to tone the skin and add volume and luster to the hair.

EPIDERMAL: or epidermis. The outer most layer of the skin. Essential oil: Plant material steam distilled to produce an oil containing concentrated healing properties of plants. May also be extracted though a chemical process. Steam distilled is best for topical use.

EXFOLIANT: A substance that sluffs off dead skin cells and helps even out skin tone.

EXTRACT: Most common being pure vanilla, coconut, banana, orange, lemon, etc. Helps to condition the skin and add a pleasant aroma to the finished product at the same time.

FRAGRANCE OIL: Fake reproduction of a flower, fruit or plant aroma. Sometimes containing a small amount of real plant matter. Not indicated for therapeutic use.

HENNA: Lawsonia alba When ground into a fine powder it can be used for many applications such as hair colorant, nail tint, paste for mehndi etc. Very conditioning to the skin.

HONEY: Aids in keeping ingredients from separating and acts as a natural preservative. Holds conditioning and emollient qualities as well. Great in place of sugar in teas.

INFUSIONS: It is the process of steeping plant material in hot water to obtain the healing properties. Most common use is teas.

MILK: Can be used in wet and dry form for various skin treatments. Helps to soften and even skin. Contains vitamin A, D, and calcium.

MOISTURIZER: A substance that smoothes and softens the skin.

NERVINE: To treat or referring to the nervous system. Especially in the areas of headaches, fatigue, stress, etc.

OLIVE OIL: Great moisturizer and skin smoother. Used in formulas for the skin and hair. Suitable for most if not all skin types.

OTC: Stands for over the counter. Otherwise products that can be bought without a prescription such as aspirin, etc.

Poultice: A towel soaked in herb tea or finely minced herbs soaked in water and applied to the skin.

STRAWBERRY: Fragaria vesca A fruit that contains vitamin C which acts as an antioxidant. Helps to tone and cleanse the skin.

STEEP: To extract the healing properties from plant material through hot water.

TINCTURE: To extract the healing properties from plants using either alcohol or oil.

TONER: A element that tightens the skin and helps smooth the texture. Can also be used to remove oil and impurities from the skin.

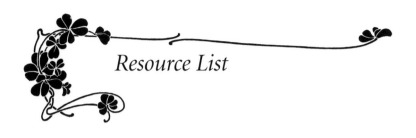

Resource List

Aromatherapy, Herb & Spice Resources

Exotic Fragrances, Inc.
1645 Lexington Avenue
New York, NY 10029 USA
Phone: (212) 410-0600
e-mail: info@exoticfragrances.com
web site: www.exoticfragrances.com

Scentsational Shoppe
945 Amsterdam Avenue
New York, NY 10025 USA
Phone: (212) 531-2007

A large number of quality fragrance oils along with charcoal for incense burning and essential oils.

InterNatural
33719 116th St.-SP
Twin Lakes , WI 53181 USA
Toll free order line: (800) 643-4221
Office phone: (414) 889-8581
Fax: (414) 889-8591
e-mail: internatural@lotuspress.com
web site: www.internatural.com

Retail mail order and internet reseller of essential oils, herbs, spices, supplements, herbal remedies, incense, books and other supplies.

Lotus Light Enterprises

P.O. Box 1008-SP
Silver Lake, WI 53170 USA
Toll free order line: (800) 548-3824
Office phone: (414) 889-8501
Fax: (414) 889-8591
e-mail: lotuslight@lotuspress.com

Wholesale distributor of essential oils, herbs, spices, supplements, herbal remedies, incense, books and other supplies. Must supply resale certificate number or practitioner license to obtain catalog of more than 10,000 items.

Incienso DeSanta Fe, Inc.

320 Headingly Ave. NW
Albuquerque, NM 87107 USA
Phone: (505) 345-0701
Native American made incense and hand crafted burners.

Aroma Medica

900 Bethlehem Pike
Erdenheim, PA 19038
Phone: (215) 233-5210 USA

Another great source of pure essential oils.

The Essential Oil Company

1719 SE Umatilla
Portland, OR 97202 USA
Phone: 1-800-729-5912
e-mail: andrew@essentialoil.com
web site: www.essentialoil.com

Essential oils, soap molds, unscented incense products, fragrance oils, glassware & more.

Herb Products Co.
11012 Magnolia Boulevard
P.O. Box 898
North Hollywood, CA 91603-0898 USA
Phone: 1-800-339-HERB or
1-800-877-3104

Very large selection of dried herbs, spices & botanicals.
Educational Courses

Johnny's Selected Seeds
1 Foss Hill Road
RR1 Box 2580
Albion, Maine 04910-9731 USA
e-mail: homegarden@johnnyseeds.com
web site: www.johnnyseeds.com

Very nice collection of herb seeds and plants.

Educational Courses

Institute for Wholistic Education

33719 116th Street
Twin Lakes, WI 53181
Phone: (414) 877-9396

Offering correspondence courses in Ayurveda

The Kevala Centre - International Yoga School

Hunsdon Road
Torquay
Devon England TQ1 1QB
Phone: +44 1803 215678
e-mail: info@kevala.co.uk
web site: www.kevala.co.uk

Excellent home study programs in Aromatherapy, Massage, Reflexology & more.

Periodicals & Publications

Lotus Press

P.O. Box 325-SP
Twin Lakes, WI 53181 USA
Toll free order line: (800) 824-6396
Office phone: (414) 889-8561
Fax: (414) 889-8591
e-mail: lotuspress@lotuspress.com
web site: www.lotuspress.com

Publisher of books in Ayurveda, aromatherpy, herbalism, alter-native modalities, spirituality and Native American studies. Extensive annotated book catalog free on request.

News from the PHARM
P.O. Box 312
Manalapan, NJ 07726 USA
e-mail: miczak@juno.com

Informative quarterly newsletter on holistic health and medical breakthroughs.

Journal of Herbs, Spices, and Medicinal Plants
10 Alice Street
Binghamton, NY 13904 USA

Aromatherapy Quarterly
P.O. Box 421
Inverness, CA 94937-0421
Fax: 415-663-9519
email: aromamag@nbn.com

Marie A. Miczak's Web-site:
http://www.angelfire.com/nj/nativetraditions

Here you can find links to learn more about courses I am teaching, articles I have written, books in print, ways of contacting me and more. Also the Distance Learning courses I offer.

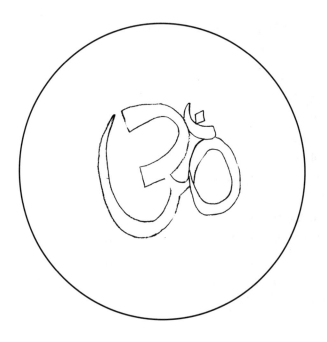

Index

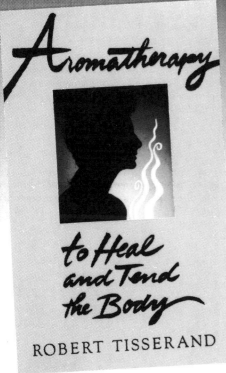

AYURVEDIC
BEAUTY CARE

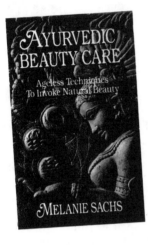

AYURVEDIC BEAUTY CARE presents both ancient and modern Ayurvedic secrests for beauty care. The aim of this book is to elevate our Western understanding of beauty to new levels with the deeper Ayurvedic insights. These insights hold powerful health promoting and enhancing methods and luxurious beauty techniques such that all levels of beauty (outer, inner, secret) can be realized in our increasingly fast-paced and chaotic world.

There are two audiences that are addressed in this volume. First and foremost, every person should be able to find what brings out their true beauty. In this light, the book is intended to be a self-care manual. At the same time, those interested in or practising as beauty therapists or aestheticians should receive the benefits of the deep insights and marvelous results Ayurveda can offer their clients.

This book represents the Ayurvedic philosophy of beauty. It includes many recipes for natural care of the skin, hair, nails, and yoga exercises for physical and mental health. It explains how to balance the constitution by using proper diet, herbs, oils, and aromas to enhance internal and external beauty. Women, in particular, will find this book very useful.

Pratima Raichur, N.D.
Founder of Tej Ayurvedic Skin Care Clinic, New York City
Creator of Bindi Skin Care

Melanie Sachs' book, *Ayurvedic Beauty Care*, is a fascinating and practical guide to using ancient techniques for enhancing good looks from the inside out. I recommend it highly.

Leslie Kenton
Author, *Joy of Beauty: A Complete Guide to Lasting Health for Today's Woman*

Ayurvedic Beauty Care is a reverent work, celebrating the fineness of the human spirit which has claimed its light.

Bri Maya Tiwari
Author, *Ayurveda: Secrets of Healing*

ISBN 0-914955-11-X   304p $17.95
PUBLISHED BY LOTUS PRESS
To order your copy, send $17.95 plus $3.00 postage and
handling ($1.50 each add'l copy) to

Lotus Press
PO Box 325
Twin Lakes, WI 53181
Request our complete book and sidelines catalog.
Wholesale inquiries welcome.

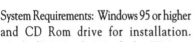

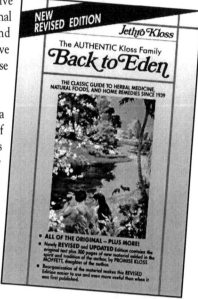

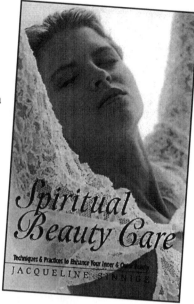

Herbs and other natural health products and information are often available at natural food stores or metaphysical bookstores. If you cannot find what you need locally, you can contact one of the follwing sources of supply.

Sources of Supply:

The following companies have an extensive selection of useful products and a long track-record of fulfillment. They have natural body care, aromatherapy, flower essences, crystals and tumbled stones, homeopathy, herbal products, vitamins and supplements, videos, books, audio tapes, candles, incense and bulk herbs, teas, massage tools and products and numerous alternative health items across a wide range of categories.

WHOLESALE:

Wholesale suppliers sell to stores and practitioners, not to individual consumers buying for their own personal use. Individual consumers should contact the RETAIL supplier listed below. Wholesale accounts should contact with business name, resale number or practitioner license in order to obtain a wholesale catalog and set up an account.

Lotus Light Enterprises, Inc.

P O Box 1008 SP
Silver Lake, WI 53170 USA
414 889 8501 (phone)
414 889 8591 (fax)
800 548 3824 (toll free order line)

RETAIL:

Retail suppliers provide products by mail order direct to consumers for their personal use. Stores or practitioners should contact the wholesale supplier listed above.

Internatural

33719 116th Street SP
Twin Lakes, WI 53181 USA
800 643 4221 (toll free order line)
414 889 8581 office phone
WEB SITE: www.internatural.com

Web site includes an extensive annotated catalog of more than 7000 products that can be ordered "on line" for your convenience 24 hours a day, 7 days a week.